T0234379

A Practical Guide to Hospital Ministry
Healing Ways

THE HAWORTH PASTORAL PRESS
Religion and Mental Health
Harold G. Koenig, MD
Senior Editor

A Practical Guide to Hospital Ministry
Healing Ways

Junietta Baker McCall, DMin

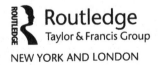

Routledge
Taylor & Francis Group

NEW YORK AND LONDON

First published 2002 by The Haworth Press, Inc.,
10 Alice Street, Binghamton, NY 13904-1580

This edition published 2015 by Routledge
711 Third Avenue New York, NY 10017
2 Park Square, Milton Park Abingdon, Oxon OX14 4RN

Routledge is an imprint of the Taylor & Francis Group, an informa business

© 2002 by The Haworth Press, Inc. All rights reserved. No part of this work may be reproduced or utilized in any form or by any means, electronic or mechanical, including photocopying, microfilm, and recording, or by any information storage and retrieval system, without permission in writing from the publisher.

TR: 8.21.03

PUBLISHER'S NOTE
The narratives presented in this book are composites and are not real stories of individuals unless otherwise indicated.

Cover design by Marylouise E. Doyle.

Library of Congress Cataloging-in-Publication Data

McCall, Junietta Baker.
    A practical guide to hospital ministry : healing ways / Junietta Baker McCall.
        p. cm.
    Includes bibliographical references and index.
    ISBN 0-7890-1211-1 (alk. paper)—ISBN 0-7890-1212-X (alk. paper)
    1. Chaplains, Hospital. 2. Church work with the sick. I.Title.

BV4335 .M29 2002
259'.411—dc21

2001045679

ISBN 13 : 978-0-7890-1212-8 (pbk)

ABOUT THE AUTHOR

Junietta Baker McCall, DMin, is Director of Pastoral Services at New Hampshire Hospital in Concord. Her previous positions include teaching in the Chicago Public School System, where she worked with developmentally challenged children, and working as Associate Pastor of the South Congregational Church in Concord. An ordained minister of the United Church of Christ, Dr. McCall has served as adjunct faculty in pastoral counseling at the Andover Newton Theological School in Newton Center, Massachusetts.

Currently, Dr. McCall supervises clergy, pastoral counseling interns, and other counseling interns who work within a holistic framework. In addition, she is a Diplomate in the American Association of Pastoral Counselors and is a licensed pastoral psychotherapist. Dr. McCall regularly conducts workshops for the United Church of Christ, New Hampshire Conference, and continues to lead workshops on aspects of grief, loss, and recovery for caregivers within the mental health system. Her recent book, *Grief Education for Caregivers of the Elderly* (Haworth), addresses the grieving issues and processes of elders and those who care for them.

CONTENTS

Acknowledgments

It is my firm conviction that hospital ministry is first and foremost a relational endeavor. Therefore, my deepest gratitude goes, first of all, to the patients and families who have opened their lives to my ministry over the past twenty years. Without their struggles and their faith, I would not have grown in wisdom and in spirit.

In addition, I am grateful to New Hampshire Hospital for providing the place and the opportunity to engage in thoughtful ministry. The hospital continues to encourage and respect a variety of reflective endeavors including the writing of this book.

A special recognition and thank-you is offered to Beverly Hospital in Beverly, Massachusetts. The Reverend Dr. John C. Pearson, Director of the Pastoral Care Department and Director/Supervisor of the Clinical Pastoral Education Program provided clinical case material and reflections from chaplain-interns. This book is much enriched by his efforts and his sharing.

To my family and colleagues I express my warmest thanks. To Bob Williams, PhD, and Harry Woodley, MDiv, I thank you for offering insight and suggestions as to the content and technical details of the manuscript. To Seth and Jeremiah McCall, I thank you for listening to my challenges, and sometimes, to my frustrations. To all those who shared their wisdom, faith, and support, thank you.

Introduction

Everyone knows that poets are born and not made in school. This is true also of painters, sculptors, and musicians. Something that is essential can't be taught; it can only be given, or earned, or formulated in a manner too mysterious to be picked apart and redesigned for the next person. (Oliver, 1994, p. 1)

A CHAPLAIN'S STORY

It is a long walk from here to there. The call comes early and it is urgent. Eleanor is dying. Could I come today? Something, I don't know what, makes me drop everything, leave the meeting early, and go to her. I mumble sounds into the air, mixed with "I'm leaving," and head out the door and up a long cement incline, my back working hard, my feet moving quickly.

The sun shines everywhere as I glimpse the remnants of a flower garden. What has happened? Five years ago it was beautiful, filled with roses and orange tiger lilies, surrounded by carefully clipped edges and newly mown grass. We used to sit there and talk as interns. I feel jarred and just a bit disappointed. They ought to be keeping the grounds better, but what did I expect? This is a state hospital. Yet, the gardens used to be so beautiful among these old buildings. "Enough of that," I chide myself. "There's no time for fussing about overgrown flower beds!"

The walk is long. It takes so much valuable time to get from here to there. Eleanor! How could it be? Two days ago she had felt better and said her depression had faded. She looked forward to living. She and I felt so much better after our last talk. How could she be dying?

Now there are two paths. Which one shall I take? The caller sounded urgent. Maybe I should go directly there. Perhaps I should get my other Bible, just in case. Do I look all right, or at least, like a pastor? I don't believe I'm saying this! Yes, best to get the Bible, but not one of those newer and fancier versions. Would she want to hear Scripture? Are there any other resources I might need? This Bible will have to do, the black one with the older words, easier to recognize and better for her memory. Now is not the time for feminist issues. Comfort is in the old, and besides, Eleanor is afraid of the new—the unknown.

Outside and down the steps, I move onward with purpose toward the brick walls. No shortcuts here, just the tried-and-true path. Speaking of symbols, I'm not male! Does she want a man or a fancy service? Goodness sakes, we share the same faith tradition! Does she want me? This is silly. I am her only pastor. She knows me and our relationship is strong and good. We had talked of hillsides and daffodils; of beautiful hymns and fear of the unknown. Hadn't she come out of her blankness last Sunday and looked at me? A smile lit her face as she received communion saying, "You're so good to me." Now that I think about it, she had been good to me too.

Almost there! The path is different today, so completely different. For one thing it's taking forever to get there. Yesterday, it was raining on this path. Someone in our group of chaplains brought forth the theory that it is wise to walk quickly in open areas and slowly under trees. Five years ago, as an intern, I would go out of my way to spend a little time in the rain as I went from place to place. It made me feel cleaner and fresher. It cleansed my spirit somehow, and helped me prepare for the pastoral care at hand.

My nose smells something comforting: hay, new-mown hay, well, not quite—but it is freshly cut grass. The mower approaches, spreading itself across the lawn with authority, a bit intimidating to say the least! Yet, with that smell, my whole being moves backward in time to the Children's Home, to Butler Hill, to Pennsylvania, to Mennonites and long hot summers with the fresh sweet smell of new-mown grass and fresh fields of golden hay waiting to be rolled and bundled for the long winters that were impossibly far from imagination's reach. Warmth spreads through my body as the images come tumbling back. It only takes a second—just a second—for summer, people, and memories to come forward from somewhere within me. I laugh.

It seems the mowing machine only moves in ovals or circles. No neat corners for this machine. Such is its essence as it rolls by throwing grass and clover over my shoes and strewing it hither and yon on the unyielding cement walk. No fussing is going on inside that machine. It only does what it can do, nothing more, nothing less. The rest, is in someone else's hands. Lucky machine!

Something falls into place inside me. I feel sure of who I am and what I do. Could that moment of sight, smell, and memory have brought such peace and resolution? "I am what I am," says the God of Old, which a professor somewhere said means God is what God causes to be. Essence and movement joined, I enter the building and move toward Eleanor's room.

She lies on the bed surrounded by the coming and going of staff. They tell her they love her and bring in other patients to say hello. They hope she is better. One patient slips and says the forbidden, "Oh, I'm sorry. You're dying." Eleanor cringes, she doesn't want to die. Does the grass or golden hay cringe when it is about to be cut? I wonder.

I lean over and give Eleanor a kiss. She is breathing in loud, raspy sounds with an oxygen tank nearby and long, forked gray tubing in her nostrils. She never could speak above a loud whisper. On purpose, or by fate, it worked well for her throughout her latter years as people had to bend down to get close enough to hear her. This was hard work for the listener but brought Eleanor closeness and bodily contact.

Eleanor and I are now alone. I ask her how she is doing. She is scared. She clenches her fist, which from past conversations means she is holding on tight, fighting to live. They still haven't told her about the cancer growing inside her body. They said it would serve no purpose. I remain unsettled over the unspoken knowledge we keep from her.

I offer the Lord's Prayer . . . the "Our Father." She says it with me. No. In truth, she says the words just ahead of me. I fumble and forget a well-known line. She moves smoothly on, leading me. Her cross is in her left hand. Gently, her fingers curl around the string. She points to it with her eyes. I'm holding her right hand and she holds on tight. It is her turn to kiss me. She does so with her hand, reaching out to put the tip of her finger gently on my nose. I laugh. I've done that to her many times as a greeting. She says, "I love you," and I say the words back. We both mean them.

Eleanor works so hard to breathe. The nurse comes in and suggests that she rest and relax. Does Eleanor know about the Do Not Resuscitate order on her chart? Has the guardian informed her of this decision that was made on her behalf? Probably not, she wants to live. She looks annoyed. Don't they know how hard she's trying? I offer to read some psalms with her. She does not indicate whether that sounds good or not, so I move ahead. Using my Bible, I read the Twenty-third Psalm. I know it from memory, but it seems emotion can halt even the best rituals and leave us speechless. I don't want to chance that again. She needs no words as she again whispers out the beloved psalm just ahead of me. The " 'Our Father' again," she rasps, and we do it again along with other psalms.

My spirit moves once more, back to the Federated Church in the small town of Harrison Valley. The sun shines once again on the highway as we walk, thirty children to town. The Children's Home must have filled both little churches in town. Bookmarks, golden stars, and ten commandment bracelets (metal and round) come to my mind's eye.

I choose three psalms I had memorized as a child. Did someone wiser than I know I would use these same verses again and again in my ministry? It is both eerie and awesome. Something startles me deep inside. My mouth and hers move almost in unison. I suggest she rest and listen, but she wants to join in. Understanding clicks within me as I realize that she feels she *must* join in. This is her life, even though these memories are mine.

I don't pray for release in the usual way. She is not ready to die. Fifteen minutes have passed, and I ask God and Eleanor to continue working. I'm speaking more to Eleanor than to God for God surely knows what to do and doesn't need my instructions. Eleanor, however, has never died before! Neither have I, but I've been with others who have been dying. That is my resource. All those people come to mind as I recall other prayers and other people. Their faces are vivid. Some held on, some were ready, and some kept their feelings to themselves.

My mind turns to Mary, a parishioner in another ministry from when I was a parish pastor. She let go as I gently gave her permission to do so. It was beautiful. In one of time's briefest moments, she came out of her near comatose condition, looked me straight in the eye, and died.

Eleanor does not want to die, and who knows, she may live any number of days or years. I am not God; I don't know. She has a right to her own wishes. So I pray that Eleanor can respond in a different way. I ask her to let God do the work. Yes, that feels and sounds right. She rests her straining neck softly on the pillow. Her eyes close gently as we continue praying.

My back is stiff; I have been holding on and praying. It dawns on me that I know I am working for Eleanor, God, the staff and the patients outside the doors, and for me. It has been good work, but it is work nevertheless. A nurse comes in to take a pulse and I use the respite to move from the bedside, out into the hall. I want to go. I want to stay. There is no urgency. I am doing what I have come to do. I move freely and talk with other patients, and read some of Eleanor's history—just in case. I am thinking of myself here; I want to be prepared for a memorial service.

How does one know when it's time to cut the grass—when its been growing too long? Silly thought! Self-admonishment enters my consciousness quickly. What is it about that grass? Even in peacefulness and assurance of heart it seems that memories are not orderly, willful things. Mine are certainly having a lively day today.

The doctor comes to the nursing station and expresses gratitude on behalf of the staff that I am there. "It's going to be a long day," he says. I ask how long. It's just something to say. He explains her medical condition and says he has no crystal ball. He feels some discomfort whenever he has to notify the family of her condition. She could die or live. He speaks of the family and the rift between Eleanor and her nearest child, a son. The son never knew how to handle Eleanor's condition. They aren't close. He asks if I will be nearby to speak with the family if they come and want to talk.

It could take all day. They offer to call me if there are any changes in Eleanor's condition, but something makes me want to stay just a little while longer. I go back into the room and assure other staff to feel free to come and go. I want them to have their private time with Eleanor too. There seems to be some relief that I am with her and they can go about tending other patients while remaining nearby.

Eleanor's head is hot now, so I move a wet washcloth back and forth over her forehead—holding her hand. I begin to sing. "Beautiful hymns" are what Eleanor wanted at her memorial service. Her whispered voice comes back to me as I recall our last talk. "Be-au-ti-ful hymns" she had said, drawing out the word *beautiful,* working it into her eyes and onto her tongue, listening with glee as her ears heard what she was saying. So I begin with the standbys that I knew she knew too: "Abide with Me," "In the Garden," and "Rock of Ages."

"Rock of ages, cleft for me, Let me hide myself in thee. Let the water and the blood . . . ." Eleanor's raspy breathing stops and her body bolts gently several times. I can no longer hear her breathing but I keep on singing. The time is 11:20. No need to call anyone. She could be resting. She has probably died. Holding her hand, I continue singing softly. Another staff person comes in and I can see she wants to be close to Eleanor so I invite her to take Eleanor's hand. It's turning blue. I walk quietly out the door to find the nurse and tell her that Eleanor has died.

The peace and quiet are over. There is work to be done. Staff feel close to one another and feel good about this gentle and loving way of dying. Patients hear the news and respond in different ways. Some cannot grasp what has occurred; still they are told one by one. It has been about an hour—that's all—about an hour.

Picking up my coat and my Bible, I leave the ward and the patients in the cafeteria having lunch. Out into the sun, I smell the newly mown grass once again. I sing to myself, "Be not afraid; I go before thee always. Come follow me and I will give thee rest."

BEGINNING ASSUMPTIONS

In the winter of 1985 I began my first job as a chaplain. I had previous clinical pastoral education experiences in three different hospital settings. I had interned in a 1,000-bed eldercare state hospital in Massachusetts, in a Catholic-run general hospital, also in Massachusetts, and at New Hampshire Hospital, a state-run psychiatric facility. I had also just finished five years of parish ministry, which of course included weekly hospital visits.

I was interviewed by the New Hampshire Council of Churches for a part-time chaplain's position on a cold day toward the end of January. A week later, I was hired by the state of New Hampshire as a chaplain in the Youth Development Center in Manchester. I don't recall receiving a written job description to go along with a brief orientation to the state's detention facility for children and adolescents.

On my first day of work, I was shown to my office—a small room on the second floor of the administration building. There was no sign on the door. The room held one small, student-size, metal desk and an ancient desk chair. There was not one piece of paper in the room. There were no files, brochures, nor any other sign of pastoral care services in the room. However, I was told that there was a part-time Roman Catholic chaplain on staff and I knew that my title was Protestant Chaplain. I was hired to work twenty hours per week.

Later, I discovered there was a huge freestanding church on the grounds. It was in this church that I found the Catholic priest and Mass. There was no doubt that the church was Catholic territory.

I wondered where I fit into the organization, and I was unprepared for the lack of resources and direction. As a result of my struggle to come to grips with this new job, I began to ask the cottage staff, children, and adolescents detained at this facility. I was told that Protestant chaplains held services in each cottage and made pastoral care visits. One cottage was used to having an informal Sunday service and the Catholic priest conducted Mass once a week in the church.

The work requirements and expectations of services turned out to be minimal. Although I stayed in this setting for only six months, it left a deep impression on my ministry. This impression remained with me as I moved to full-time chaplaincy in a state-run psychiatric hospital.

Why a Book on Hospital Ministry?

Sixteen years later, I still think of that small office with no paper, no files, no brochures, and no sign on the door. I think of my eighteen years of training and work in hospital ministry. In that time, I have observed the strengths and complexities of hospital ministry firsthand. I have also experienced emotional highs and lows and am tuned in to the wear and tear that this form of ministry has on those engaged in it over a period of time.

During the last few years, I have paid closer attention to my colleague's expressions of concern about the care and funding of this type of ministry as well as their feelings of being burdened by changes in the health care field. I've witnessed the increasing brevity of hospitalization time and the rising severity of health care issues and needs during the course of hospitalization. Many of these changes have left chaplains feeling much like compassionate dinosaurs moving through someone else's virtual reality!

Why, then, a book on hospital ministry? The most passionate answer is that we need to let people know who we are and what we do. This is so crucial to the growth and development of hospital ministry, for in many ways, hospital ministry continues to be an undervalued, misunderstood, and underused resource in the health care and pastoral ministry field.

Some of the lack of use, value, and understanding of hospital ministry can be attributed to the manner in which clergy and chaplains are trained; the ways in which pastoral care departments are involved in the organizational systems of both hospital processes and church ministry; the sometimes negative perceptions medical/clinical staff have of clergy as unhelpful in the hospital setting; and the need for research, practical journal contributions, and comprehensive books by trained and mature chaplains in the field.

This call to share the practical knowledge of the nuts and bolts of hospital ministry was recently reinforced by a colleague who has been a clinical pastoral educator for twenty-two years. When asked what books he used for the training of his students in hospital ministry, his response was, "There is no comprehensive guide to hospital ministry available. There are just bits and pieces." Furthermore, he stated that he would be very pleased to have access to a comprehensive and practical guide to hospital ministry and said that his students complained regularly about the lack of such a resource.

HOSPITAL MINISTRY AS HEALTH CARE RESOURCE

Every professional discipline needs resources to assist their members in the struggle to keep themselves and others informed about best theories and practices. In this respect, hospital ministry is no different from other health care professions. But, unlike some professions, we continue to struggle, and perhaps resist, putting our theories and practices into an organized form that establishes clearly what we do and how we do it.

The purpose of this book is to further the task of consolidating information on what hospital chaplains do. In taking on this task, it is hoped that this work will become a resource to individuals engaged in hospital ministry. In addition, the information found in this book is intended to be helpful to hospital administrators, educators, and persons seeking to provide spiritual and pastoral resources to hospitalized individuals and their families.

To accomplish these purposes, this book will assume the need for a purposeful, pragmatic, meaningful, integrated, and systemic view of hospital ministry. In addition, chaplains and educators will be encouraged to support an even greater shift to a knowledge and skill-based ministry that both incorporates and goes beyond current training approaches in the field. The motivation for such a shift can still be found in the basic "call" and response to pastoral care and hospital ministry. This motivational "call" has always involved the desire to be with those who are ill and in distress and to help those who are healing and moving toward recovery. Such a call is naturally embedded in, and supported by, all processes that focus on quality care and empowerment through holistic and spiritually enhanced practices. To this end, hospital ministry has identifiable outcomes of its services and has the potential of being an even greater resource to the health care field.

Too often, what has been taught in clinical programs is "how to do a pastoral visit," and, "how to provide crisis-supportive interventions." These are essential first steps in hospital ministry, but are incomplete by themselves, and may lead to fragmented services. In today's health care and specialized ministry services, education and training must be progressive and thorough. They must include experiences that increase one's expertise in working with individuals, groups, families, consumers, and systems. These services must be integrated into the total structure and resources of hospitals at all levels of mission, philosophy, and program.

Furthermore, not only is the integration of hospital ministry into the fabric of hospital foundations in need of repair and reformulating, but hospital ministry must also strive to be a resource to the larger community and the Church. This is quite a task to undertake, for the larger community and the Church appear to have limited ideas of how to use twenty-first century chaplaincy as a resource, nor have many congregations completed their struggle to come to a practical consensus about their own "call" to be engaged in hospital ministry. To this end, it can be said that the integration of hospital ministry into the structure and resources of church life is often absent, elusive, and fragmented in many churches. Where this is so, a reformulation of ministry to the sick and hospitalized is needed.

This book is offered as a resource for clergy, pastoral and spiritual care providers, hospitals, and churches with the goal of helping hospital ministry grow as a resource to individuals and organizations. It will help in several ways. First, the material covered in this text provides a benchmark for establishing hospital ministries and for reviewing current programs. Second, the material found in these pages could be used as a means for advocacy for professionals in the field, for patients, and for the larger community. This book is also intended to further the general process of communication and dialogue about hospital ministry. Finally, it is meant to be a resource for the creation, and in some places strengthening, of bridges toward increased integration of hospital ministry in secular and sacred organizations where support and understanding of hospital ministry is weak or nonexistent.

TAKING THE TEMPERATURE OF HOSPITAL MINISTRY

In the behavioral health care field, it is considered crucial to determine an individual's current functioning level. Otherwise, one is in danger of either going backward or forward too quickly, and expecting too much! To determine an individual's current level of functioning, one asks the individual to perform certain functions and records the results. If a change is needed or wanted, the current level of functioning is compared to past levels or current standards and expectations. Improvement is accomplished in a planned way through practicing certain behaviors and engaging in regular assessments.

Example

Just before heart valve surgery, John breathed into an Iso Sporometer and attained the measurement of 3,500 ml. After his surgery he was able to reach only about 1,000 ml with some hard work on the part of his lungs, heart, and chest. He practiced breathing into this machine every day. Each day, for two weeks, he raised the numbers that represented his current functioning level in the area of breathing. On the thirteenth day after his surgery he was again able to attain the level of 3,500 ml. He felt successful, having achieved his goal of returning to his previous level of functioning. A similar process was used to pay attention to John's weight, fluid retention, and temperature. The struggle was to have his new "current level of functioning" become as good as it could be.

In the next few pages, the current level of functioning of hospital ministry is described. These descriptions are generalizations based on practice, research, and professional dialogue occurring in the field today. For the purposes of this book, hospital ministry's current level of functioning is described by paying attention to its strengths and needs. As you read these pages, you may wish to use this review as a way of measuring your ministry.

GROWING NEEDS IN THE FIELD
OF HOSPITAL MINISTRY

While it can be said that the needs of hospital ministry are numerous, and that some of these needs are idiosyncratic to specific situations, some are universal. Six such universal needs come to the foreground in any discussion of hospital ministry:

1. A paradigm shift
2. Training and education
3. Hospital systems integration and advocacy
4. Integration within churches
5. Enhanced community integration
6. Increased link with other spiritual traditions

The Need for a Paradigm Shift

By speaking of hospital ministry as a health care resource, I am intentionally challenging those in the health care and spiritual care fields to make a paradigm shift. This shift involves a movement away from being undervalued, misunderstood, and underused toward being better understood, more valued, and of greater use. This is a challenge for the field as a whole, even though there are people, programs, and agencies that are highly valued, understood, and used well. Often, however, hospital ministry is met with ups and downs, and frequently, with ambivalence.

At New Hampshire Hospital, for example, sometimes the department of pastoral services appears to be a true and valued member of the health care team. There are also times when it is forgotten and even blocked from doing its work. It is seldom the case that churches and their members understand what the department and its chaplains do. Every now and then someone says, or implies, that chaplaincy and pastoral counseling aren't real ministry. Many times the department has received glowing feedback from patients, families, colleagues, and persons of high responsibility in the hospital and health care system.

To further hospital ministry and create the desired paradigm value shift, we first need to engage in strenuous self-reflection and increased self-valuing within our field. We need to see hospital ministry as a valued and useful resource for all persons and agencies, and be able to talk about and demonstrate what we do. Also, we need to share the effects and outcomes of what we do in ways that others can understand and more easily integrate into preferred health care practices.

The Need for Training and Education

Hospital ministry once belonged to community clergy who were interested and willing to make visits to hospitalized persons from their congregations. Those who found this type of work rewarding were often moved to visit strangers also. Often, they saw this visitation as part of a mission or mandate for compassion and to help the needy. In more recent years, a cadre of professionals who have taken clinical pastoral education coursework and/or have advanced clinically in pastoral counseling have been added to the hospital ministry field. More recently, individuals who (through personal experience, lay ministry training programs, and spiritual and nonreligious focus) have found placement in hospital ministry based on the growing interest in spiritual concerns and more private, individualized aspects of spirituality.

This growing diversity within the field has led to an increased need for a body of practical resources. In the past, standards and resources were passed to future generations through training and education. A place and process for identity formation was also present. Now, the need for unified educational and training standards is even greater. These resources, however, will not replicate the past. Furthermore, the partnerships needed to create these resources will need to be creative and inventive if they are to succeed.

The Need for Hospital Systems Integration and Advocacy

In the state of New Hampshire we have a grassroots, loosely committed organization of hospital chaplains. We meet now and then to be supportive and act as resources for each other. Mostly we discuss how to present our profession to the hospitals in which we are located, and we wonder with great anxiety about the downsizing of funds and personnel within our agencies and departments. All of us shake our puzzled heads when issues of hospital accreditation, scope of services, quality improvement projects, competencies, and other common expectations in today's health care field are mentioned.

These things were never part of the training that individuals received on their journey to become chaplains. Furthermore, the processes and changes required are difficult for some colleagues to pick up on the job. Yet, the need to learn health care language and processes is crucial if we are to be a growing resource to patients and organizations alike.

The Need for Integration Within Churches

Most ordained chaplains and persons from religious orders are ecclesiastically endorsed to engage in hospital ministry. They are also ordained or commissioned in some way to work on behalf of the Church. Part of the difficulty with the current process is that a church may send forth people who want to be chaplains, but it does not necessarily encourage or initiate such action, nor does it appear to know how to consistently relate to chaplains while they are in the field.

Example

New Hampshire Hospital, in Concord, New Hampshire, has had chaplains since 1856. Prior to that time, between 1842 and 1856, there were churches in the town of Concord that received psychiatric patients into their church communities on Sundays. As times and treatments changed, community clergy began to visit patients on hospital grounds and eventually began having services at the hospital.

Modern treatment and advanced technologies will continue to challenge parish clergy and churches who have not yet come to grips with how they relate to specialized ministries outside the Church's established walls of mortar and brick. As current technology changes and resources become more limited, hospital ministries may not have the luxury of being distantly related to the Church's ministry. Therefore, chaplains need to intentionally reach out to the Church and faith community now, if they have not done so before. In addition, spiritual resource communities need to reach out to chaplains if they are to survive and if the Church is to be a people of compassion and caring for all. Churches and congregations that have not yet established hospital ministry priorities will need to find ways of engaging in this mission, including ways to train volunteers, visitors, and ministers. Such parish-based training has grown through the years and would greatly benefit from the expertise of chaplains in the health care field.

The Need for Enhanced Community Integration

Recently, health care has adopted a general stance of providing "seamless services." These services focus on the many and varied health care needs that occur throughout a person's life. Seamless services are based on these needs rather than on discrete, separate locales where services are provided. For an organization such as a hospital, the concept of "seamless services" leaves them struggling to view themselves as a building with no walls.

In addition, the practicalities of providing services—i.e., training and past experiences of current staff; and the expectations of patients and their families—make seamless services difficult to put into practice. To meet these needs, hospitals have placed greater emphasis on departments of care and community integration and on indicators of community communication and collaboration. Although some pastoral care and chaplaincy departments may be used to working closely with community clergy and volunteers—and may even be providing clinical training for these persons—the fullness of seamless pastoral services and community integration has yet to be tapped in hospital ministry.

The Need for an Increased Link with Other Spiritual Traditions

Hospital ministry in the United States has historically consisted of pastoral care by ordained persons of Roman Catholic, Protestant, and Jewish faiths. This long and cherished tradition worked fairly well in a country consisting predominately of these three traditions. However, the spiritual face of America is neither limited nor confined to organized spiritual traditions that are neatly lumped into a handful of categories. We need to address this spiritual and religious plurality within ourselves and consider possible changes implied by the diversity of hospitalized individuals in need of pastoral care.

CURRENT STRENGTHS OF HOSPITAL MINISTRY

The strengths of hospital ministry as a vocation and specialized ministry are numerous, and different aspects are likely to be highlighted in each individual situation. However, the development and integration of hospital ministry within the medical/clinical organization of the hospital service system has been greatly enhanced by the following strengths:

- A mission-mandate fulfilled
- A person-centered approach
- The spiritual part of mind, body, and spirit
- A relational-connective approach
- Involvement in multiple contexts and systems
- Competent professionals
- A process approach

A Mission-Mandate Fulfilled

Chaplains and pastoral care departments have made skilled and compassionate contributions to the health care field. These contributions have benefitted people stationed in all corners of the world. They have also benefitted persons in local community hospitals and those miles away from home in specialized hospitals receiving state of the art psychiatric care, surgical care, and services not available at local hospitals. These contributions contrast greatly to an otherwise possible "out of sight, out of mind" approach that local congregations might have used if left to their own preferences and resources.

From a chaplain's point of view, no matter what the religious or spiritual orientation, we can answer "yes" to the Christian question posed by Jesus (Matthew 25:37-39 RSV), ". . . when did we see thee hungry and feed thee, or thirsty and give thee drink? And when did we see thee a stranger and welcome thee, or naked and clothe thee? And when did we see thee sick or in prison and visit thee?" A chaplain's answer to this pastoral care question about visitation is, "daily, we visited thee."

In the Hebrew tradition of Rabbi Hillel, we can answer "yes" to the admonition to bring humane contributions to difficult situations such as hospital ministry. For, according to Hillel, "In a place where no one behaves like a human being, you must strive to be human!" (Stern, 1982, p. 19). It can be said that chaplains of all faiths strive to be faithful humans in the midst of all kinds of human despair, both internal and interpersonal.

Also, chaplains who understand and support natural, physical, mental, and spiritual interconnections can say that they, too, are involved in hospital ministry. For often a need exists to reconnect the physical body to the healthy life force of the universe. To spirit-filled mandates for love and compassion, a chaplain can agree with leaders such as Helen Nearing who writes, "Everybody can love, in the place where they are. In the physical body in which [we] are. In the life in which [we] are involved. We can all add our share of love without leaving the room" (Ryan, 1994, p. 232).

A Person-Centered Approach

Above all things, hospital ministry is a person-centered approach to ministry and health care. By definition, the focus of this type of ministry is on each individual's needs and resources for healing. For these reasons, those engaged in hospital ministry endeavor to focus on listening to people while helping them and their families assess issues pertaining to their lives such as health and illness, even dying. It is recognized by individual chaplains that some faith traditions specialize in sacramental ministry and others in ministry of Word and prayer. Still other chaplains specialize in clinical pastoral care and counseling. Nevertheless, all chaplains know and use the person-centered approach to ministry and usually specialize in this approach.

The Spiritual Part of Mind, Body, and Spirit

Chaplains also understand the essential connection of mind, body, and spirit. We understand the need for this holistic approach and work toward this end on behalf of patients and their families. A clinical psychologist friend told me recently, "Everybody these days wants a part of the spiritual component. I know psychologists who claim that by virtue of baptism they are able to provide clinical services in the area of spiritual healing. It takes more than being brought up in a church. Clinically based spiritual care takes special training and expertise just as any other component of care. That's the contribution pastoral counselors make to the field." We are aware, by virtue of call and training, that at all times our focus must include the spiritual part of mind, body, and spirit.

A Relational-Connective Approach

The nature of hospital ministry is such that chaplains often find themselves relating to a diverse group of people who, in stressful situations, may be experiencing disconnection and feelings of isolation. On many occasions, chaplains have helped people connect with God or other Higher Powers that they have found distant, wrathful, or uncaring perhaps. On many occasions, it is the chaplain who sits with a dying person. Sometimes it is a chaplain who helps ease the stress on someone who, in need of a friend, may be causing chaos and havoc with ward staff and family. It may be a chaplain who is called upon to help make connections, listen, and perhaps say things that help individuals work with their medical team and accept treatment options that otherwise seem overwhelming and unwanted.

Chaplains know they are called upon to be supportive and connective ears for the patient, family, staff, the organization, and differing belief systems. They treat this knowledge with respect knowing how important this function is for all concerned. This task of making connections, through communication, problem solving, and conflict resolution, is an important task that requires an appreciation of the complex issues people face during a course of hospitalization.

Involvement in Multiple Contexts and Systems

In hospital ministry, making connections is accomplished on many levels. Chaplains who work holistically must understand systems, multiple contexts, and the complexity of biopsychosocial and spiritual concerns of individuals and organizations. For some time, chaplains have had to learn to work in an essentially secular system while bringing sacred concepts, beliefs, and values to bear on treatment issues and processes. For chaplains, understanding the diversity of the health care system and the beliefs and values of persons in need of treatment is crucial in promoting health and healing. Most chaplains take care to learn as much as they can about the way these systems work. They are usually highly motivated to use these systems to promote wellness within organizations and individuals.

Competent Professionals

In a previous paragraph, I referred to a growing need for hospital ministry personnel to be trained to a greater degree in the administrative, structural, and philosophical underpinnings of this kind of ministry. At the same time, the competency of most chaplains, as it pertains to pastoral care (and sometimes, to pastoral counseling), is of the highest quality. These competent professionals strengthen the field of hospital ministry and give it internal integrity as well as status among other health care disciplines.

A Process Approach

Most chaplains have been clinically trained to reflect on processes. These reflections vary depending on the stance, style, and training of each individual chaplain. However, most clinical pastoral traditions encourage the use of process methods as well as person-centered approaches to healing and recovery. The action-reflection process helps the chaplain gather insight into his or her functioning as chaplain. The processes or dynamics of persons, relationships, and systems, help chaplains understand patterns and behaviors that may be involved in processes of healing and illness for persons and families. Also, the willingness to analyze processes within oneself helps the spiritual care provider know his or her strengths and limitations and to plan care interventions accordingly.

THE INTERACTIVE FORMAT OF THIS BOOK

In this time of growing technological sophistication, the reader of any book must be engaged in multiple ways if he or she is to be motivated to read and learn. This is particularly true of those involved in initial training but also true of those who have practiced in a given field for some time. As one clinical pastoral intern stated to her supervisor, "Couldn't you redo this student's handbook in sound bites? I'm not used to reading lengthy paragraphs!" One might say that this is a typical viewpoint of many people in the twenty-first century—the age of the Internet. Make learning work for me!

In formatting this book, every attempt has been made to provide opportunities for readers to be engaged in thinking about hospital ministry. To this end, the book focuses primarily on the standards and practices of hospital ministry as it is likely to be found in numerous hospital settings.

The reader is encouraged to consider his or her own ministry and to participate in activities suggested in various chapters. The reader's engagement in self-reflection and assessment is accomplished through the use of:

- Case material
- Opportunities to reflect on personal experience
- Opportunities to use continuous quality improvement principles
- Worksheets and questionnaires

The Use of Case Material

Throughout the book, the reader will find vignettes, stories, and poetry, the content of which expresses some aspect of hospital ministry. These vignettes enhance the standards and practices of hospital ministry. The narratives (stories and poetry) presented are composites of experiences and are in no way meant to be actual stories of individuals unless otherwise indicated.

Opportunities to Reflect on Experience

It is the nature of all practical guides to encourage readers to compare and contrast what is presented with the reader's own experiences. This is a good technique that can be accomplished in numerous ways. Some will find it helpful to write in the margins, take notes, or undertake some sort of journaling process. Department members may find it helpful to set aside time for discussion of the material presented.

Opportunities to Use Continuous Quality Improvement Principles

"State-of-the-art" health care is best represented in the twenty-first century by a focus on continuous quality improvement of services. Continuous quality improvement, as presented in this book, is a tool that has become fairly universal in health care. However, this tool is more prevalent in health care institutions than it is in pastoral and spiritual care programs. Because this current trend in hospitals is a helpful tool, readers will be encouraged to use it in assessing their own ministries. The tool is most clearly presented in the development of vision, mission, and goals, and is implied throughout the book.

Worksheets and Questionnaires

Finally, the use of worksheets and questionnaires is encouraged throughout the book. In some cases these materials are provided within a chapter and on other occasions they are included in the Appendixes. These materials may be copied and used as needed.

AN OVERVIEW

Chapter 1, "Introduction to Ministry in Hospital Settings," focuses on understanding specialized hospital ministries and notes how these ministries have changed. Early traditional ministries, newer clinical traditions, and more recent spiritual care directions are described. Current specializations are considered by focusing on defining criteria for each specialization, training sources, services provided, skill attainment and patients served. This focus on spiritual care providers and chaplains helps the reader understand the increasing diversity in the field of hospital ministry. In addition, the wide range of skills, services, and connections of these caregivers lends itself to further considerations about the challenges and changes in the field of hospital ministry.

Chapter 2, "Understanding Hospitalization Process and Patient Needs," offers a health care service wheel as a means of looking at health care in the twenty-first century. Changes in hospitalization and care are also noted. The service wheel and changes in hospitalization and health care provide a context for subsequent information on what patients want. Since it is crucial for all health care providers to understand what patients want and need during the course of hospitalization, the rest of the chapter consists of a summary of recent research in this area. This research is obtained from general hospitals, psychiatric, and specialized settings. The chapter concludes with a list of suggested ways of determining what parents want and need from a chaplain.

Chapter 3, "Health, Healing, Illness, and Recovery" sets forth practical questions and discussion concerning broad themes of health and illness, wellness and recovery, and healing and hope. Concepts and experiences about these themes are often complex but essential to recovery. By focusing on core images in any of these areas, chaplains and patients may find clues to facilitating positive treatment outcomes. Some core health images are presented constructively, while others are considered challenging and potentially destructive. Knowing how to assess these images will assist spiritual care providers and consumers of health care services.

In Chapter 4, the focus on providers and consumers shifts to the task of establishing a vision and a mission for hospital ministry. The models provided for developing a vision of hospital ministry are both practical and inspiring. Specific tools used for establishing vision and mission statements are borrowed directly from new management theories with further references provided in the bibliography. Exercises are provided throughout the chapter to help readers follow along and create their own value, vision, and ministry statements.

Since chaplains and students often wonder about the "how tos" of hospital ministry, and may have difficulty finding such material in a compact and useful form, Chapter 5 provides a practical guide for integrating professional needs into the practice of hospital ministry. This chapter describes the fundamentals of chaplaincy and is a good brush-up chapter. It presents some material that may be new to readers, whether they are newcomers or veterans in the field. The chapter ends with an exercise titled, "Identifying Professional Ministry Needs."

"Developing Caring Contexts for Health and Healing," Chapter 6, puts forward a core assumption of this book—that the patient is both patient and healer. Although this concept is not totally original, it has yet to gain practical momentum in the field. In this chapter the term "context" is used to refer to people, places, and processes, thus the patient-healer and spiritual care provider are considered essential people-contexts for healing. Care-based processes and places provide additional, caring contexts for healing. Finally, relationships are discussed as essential contexts for healing. In each case, caring contexts for healing are discussed in ways that lead to more effective hospital ministry.

Chapter 7, "Focusing on Skill Development," breaks down basic pastoral care practices into manageable, functional strategies and processes. Chaplains and spiritual care providers are encouraged to use common sense and engage in commonly accepted practices such as making initial contacts; providing practical help; being supportive; offering brief counseling; and providing effective crisis intervention.

In Chapter 8, "Going Beyond the Basics," eight areas of advanced hospital ministry that require both experience and further training are discussed. Some of the training required can be in the form of self-education while other training will involve more formal endeavors. Areas included are administration, consultation, ethics, advanced pastoral care, pastoral counseling, teaching and supervision, research and writing, and interpretation and advocacy within the wider community. After reading this chapter, the reader will be encouraged to develop a professional plan for growth and development.

The final chapter, "Making Connections," uses systemic and team concepts to speak to important issues of integrating hospital ministries into hospital organizations; the wider community; in the work of community clergy; clergy consultants; and within church life. These connections help us accomplish our vision and mission, and are our resources for helping us do the work we do while reaping the potential rewards this type of ministry can offer.

Chapter 1

Introduction to Ministry in Hospital Settings

Sometimes situations come along in our lives that give birth to compassion. But one can also be more deliberate. Intentionally placing oneself in situations where people are struggling and need help, and being present to that experience, can be transformative. . . . What matters for this means of transformation is letting the life circumstances of others move one's heart. (Borg, 1998, p. 127)

Recently, as I began thinking about this first chapter of the book, I spent the better part of a week trying to identify the various names, affiliations, types of training, and focus of services for persons engaged in hospital ministry. I was surprised to settle on thirteen categories to include in this chapter. Once these categories were chosen, it was a logical step to group them into larger categories, and then into three major classifications of traditional ministries, newer traditions, and recent directions. The newer traditions were further divided into two sections: clinical pastoral education and clinical pastoral counseling (see Tables 1.1-1.4).

This categorization of people, functions, skills, and services is intended to bring increased clarity to a field that is becoming more diverse. The increased categories of hospital ministry have brought new directions and challenges that are discussed later in this chapter. In efforts to use this information, readers may wish to reflect on their own ministries and the challenges faced. For those who wish to review their ministry or department using this format, a blank form is provided in Appendix A.

TABLE 1.1. Hospital Ministries, Traditional

Name	Defining Criteria	Training Source	Service Delivered	Competencies	Patients Served
1. Parish Pastors Priests Rabbis	Ordination vows Relation/Call to serve local church or congregation	Theological schools Bible colleges	Visits Support Prayer Sacraments Ordinances Referrals Education Resources	May include: One or more units of clinical pastoral education or equivalent. Field education experience. Experience in hospital visitation. Continuing education hours. Experience in local church(s).	Members of own faith community
2. Chaplains	All of the above plus: hired by hospital and possibly endorsed by faith group.	All of the above plus: perhaps connected to any of a number of chaplain's organizations.	All of the above plus: worship, memorial services, family/staff support, team and organizational involvement, focused visits, counseling, crisis intervention, documentation of services.	All of the above plus: experience in hospitals as chaplains. Focused coursework relating to hospital ministry.	Patients from variety of locations and faith traditions
3. Pastoral/ Religious Consultants	Ordination/vows Relation/call to serve church or congregation Perhaps stipend by hospital	Same as above	Same as parish pastor	Same as parish pastor	Patients from own denomination or faith tradition

TABLE 1.2. Hospital Ministries, Newer Traditions: Clinical Pastoral Education

Name	Defining Criteria	Training Source	Service Delivered	Competencies	Patients Served
4. Clinical Pastoral Chaplains	Ordained, Religious, and lay persons with ecclesiastical endorsement for Chaplaincy. Hired by hospital.	Theological schools and/or religious studies plus several (4) clinically supervised educational experiences.	Same as 1 and 2	Same as 1 and 2 plus possible membership in clinical pastoral organization. Clinical method of service delivery. Function at advanced clinical level.	Patients from a variety of locations and faith traditions
5. Pastoral Care Educators	Supervisor/member of recognized clinical pastoral organization	Theological school and/or religious studies. Clinical pastoral supervisory training.	Same as 1 and 2 plus provides training program, students, supervision, educational events, educational advocacy	Numerous units of clinical pastoral education. Focused coursework on supervision and adult learning theory. Credentialed by clinical pastoral organization as educator.	May include same patient contact as above, plus provision of indirect patient care through supervision of students
6. Clinical Pastoral Education Students	Usually endorsed by ecclesiastical body for training program	Varies: may have high school diploma, Associate's degree, college degree, be in a theological school, be a parish pastor, or desire to become an educator.	Includes the learning and practice of 1 and 2 at varying levels from introductory to advanced. May include introductory to advanced supervisory training.	Determined by standards set by recognized clinical pastoral education organization as evidenced by learning contracts, and evaluations at end of each clinical pastoral unit, and by advancement at regional and national levels.	Same as 1

TABLE 1.3. Hospital Ministries, Newer Traditions: Clinical Pastoral Counseling

Name	Defining Criteria	Training Source	Service Delivered	Competencies	Patients Served
7. Clinical Pastoral Chaplains	Same as 4	Theological schools and/or religious studies plus minimum of one clinically supervised educational experience, plus additional clinically supervised counseling experiences.	Same as 1 and 2. In addition may provide pastoral counseling, lead therapy groups, and provide primary pastoral psychotherapy in conjunction with team and treatment plans.	Often the same as 1 and 2 plus: membership and certification in recognized pastoral counseling organization. May be certified or licensed by the state in which services are provided. Advanced use of clinical method for delivery of care and counseling services.	Same as 2 plus: persons referred for pastoral counseling, group counseling, and/or pastoral psychotherapy.
8. Pastoral Care Educators	Same as 1 plus: ordained clergy or chaplains with relation and call to serve church or congregation.	Theological schools, bible colleges, experience in church or religious organizations. Has taken supervised pastoral care specialist program from recognized pastoral counseling organization.	Focuses on assessment, diagnosis, brief counseling interventions, referral, and resources for further therapy and/or health care services.	Same as 1, may include 2 or 3, plus added competencies in supportive counseling and referral.	Usually same as 1 if parish based, or 2 if chaplaincy based.
9. Pastoral Counselors and Pastoral Psychotherapists	Usually endorsed by church or congregation membership and certification by rec-	Graduate and post graduate degree work in theological studies, counseling, and psycho-	May include same as 1, 2, 7, and 8, plus includes therapeutic caseload at advanced level.	Determined by standards set by recognized clinical pastoral counseling organization	Requested by patient Identified by pastoral counselor, and/or team referred.

Name	Defining Criteria	Training Source	Service Delivered	Competencies	Patients Served
	ognized clinical pastoral counseling organization; may be certified or licensed by state.	therapy, or similar clinical fields. Advanced training in pastoral counseling and pastoral psychotherapy.		and state health care licensing and certification boards. Advanced level of functioning.	
10. Pastoral Counseling Educators	Supervisor-diplomate in recognized pastoral counseling organization or fellow under supervision of supervision.	Same as 9, plus advanced training and practice in clinical supervision of pastoral care and counseling students.	In addition to pastoral care and counseling work listed under 1 and 2, educator also provides training program, students, supervision, educational events, and educational advocacy.	Numerous units of pastoral counseling, internships, and residencies. Focused coursework on supervision and adult learning theory. Credentialed by clinical pastoral counseling organization as diplomate or fellow under supervision of diplomate.	May include same patient contact as 2, 7, and 9, plus provision of indirect patient care and counseling through supervision of pastoral counseling students.
11. Counseling Interns and Residents	Usually endorsed by ecclesiastical body for training program or part of educational internship focusing on holistic counseling methods.	Graduate and postgraduate clinical pastoral and counseling degree programs.	Includes the learning and practice of 7 and 9 at varying levels from introductory to advanced May include introductory to advanced supervision of counseling.	Standards set by recognized clinical pastoral counseling organization as evidenced by learning contracts and evaluations, and by advancement at state, regional, and national levels.	Same as 7 and 9

TABLE 1.4. Hospital Ministries: Recent Directions: Postmodern Spirituality

Name	Defining Criteria	Training Source	Service Delivered	Competencies	Patients Served
12. Spiritual Care Chaplain	Spiritual care chaplain may use religious or God language and have wide definition of what is spiritual.	May have background from a theological school, hospice training, spiritual direction, retreats, and conferences.	Visits, support, varied resources, referrals.	May have experience in spiritual care training programs. Usually has college degree and perhaps further education.	Same as 2
13. Persons with Holistic Focus	Mind-body-spirit focus with or without traditional religious connections.	Professionals with training in other than religious or pastoral field. Additional training in variety of spiritual practices, beliefs, and treatment.	Usually part of services provided under other disciplines, such as: nursing, psychology, social services, medical services, and rehabilitation services.	May include coursework as part of training for primary discipline. May include continuing education and advanced training.	Same as 2. Patients are those accessing services of department or discipline in which provider is credentialed.

TRADITIONAL MINISTRIES

Parish Pastors, Priests, Rabbis, and Others

Clergy who view hospital ministry as visitation of the sick are included under traditional ministries, as Table 1.1 illustrates. Visitation is offered as part of one's clerical duties, or as a self-chosen interest. This category consists of parish pastors, priests, rabbis and persons of religious orders. This is a large category since leaders from most major religions undertake hospital visitation when someone from their own faith community is hospitalized.

Since Jewish and Christian biblical times, visitation of the sick has been an expectation of family and community members, churches, and congregations. Quite early on, the role of visitation was also assigned

.

to compassionate and willing deacons and elders. As hospitals came into being, patients were often moved from home to hospitals when illness fell upon them. Clergy were then given the task of visiting sick members of their congregations in the hospital. This visitation continued, even in situations where lay visitors and elders made hospital calls. Today, community clergy continue to provide the bulk of visitation and spiritual care services in many hospital settings where patients associated with their faith communities are hospitalized.

Chaplains

Many hospitals today have a long-standing tradition of providing chaplains who meet job expectations as established by individual hospitals. These requirements are often influenced by established standards of specific faith groups such as ordination and/or ecclesiastical endorsement. Some of these chaplains may also rely on "on the job" training in their new positions.

Example

At New Hampshire Hospital, an acute care psychiatric facility, the transition to hiring community clergy to provide services to hospitalized patients took place by 1856. Prior to this time patients were often free to attend worship services in the town of Concord. As treatment styles changed, the patients were less free to move from the hospital to the community on a daily basis. Thus, community clergy-chaplains brought these essential services to the hospital. Visits were conducted and worship services were held in an auditorium, and later, were held in a full-size chapel in the main hospital building.

Right through the 1950s, chaplains lived on hospital grounds and provided services day and night. Having chaplains on staff meant greater availability of services to persons throughout the state of New Hampshire who were often far away from their regular faith communities, and, through choice and the vicissitudes of isolative events that often come with mental illness, were no longer connected to faith traditions in their hometowns. All of these factors led to growth in the tradition of providing Protestant, Catholic, and Jewish chaplains at this hospital. An interesting by-product of these changes was the growing number of patients and former patients who no longer identified with a specific Catholic, Protestant, or Jewish congregation, but rather with the hospital chapel and ministry.

Pastoral/Religious Consults

Another category of clergy who provide hospital ministry came into being partly as a result of the use of paid chaplaincy services. Although hospital chaplains at that time were accountable to their churches and hospitals, they were usually Protestant, Catholic or Jewish. Still, many faith traditions had no specific representation in hospital chaplaincy services. To serve these patients, chaplains needed to broaden their perspectives and focus of their services, and determine when it would be essential to bring in consults from other specific faith groups. Often these pastoral/religious consults would be Mormon elders, Orthodox priests, or clergy from other church traditions such as Christian Scientists or Seventh-Day Adventists. Consults were provided on voluntary and reimbursed bases. The focus of their service was narrow, and consisted of responding to specific referrals. In situations and times when communities had clergy who were willing to engage in crisis services, the consult service went smoothly. When clergy were not willing to take referrals nor engage in this form of hospital ministry to nonparishioners, difficulties would often be experienced by the hospital, chaplains, and patients.

Traditional Ministries Today

The defining criteria for traditional ministries today remain ordination or vows of clergy/chaplains who are engaged in hospital ministry and their relation to specific churches and congregations. Sources of training often include theological school and perhaps religious orders for those who have taken vows of service. Services provided are generally supportive and pastoral, and may include worship and sacraments or provision of ordinances. These traditional hospital chaplains, or consults, are deemed competent if they serve a church, have some experience in hospital ministry, and perhaps some clinical pastoral education, which is valued and available. Competency in this form of ministry is based on a church credentialing process.

NEWER TRADITIONS

Clinical Pastoral Education

Newer traditions in hospital ministry are listed in Tables 1.2 and 1.3. These ministries grow out of two types of clinical training and two service foci. The first professional style and affiliation comes from advanced training known as clinical pastoral education. These groups are traced back to the experiences and use of trained chaplains begun by Anton Boison, who was hospitalized with a mental illness in the early part of the twentieth century.

In this clinical pastoral care training model, students and chaplains use clinical methods of learning and provide pastoral care services based primarily on an action-reflection process. A focus on the developing identity of the pastoral person is integral to the training process. Training also includes mastering the ability to define presenting problems; noting biopsychosocial and spiritual histories; assessing individual needs; and developing pastoral care plans.

Clinical Pastoral Chaplains

Chaplains trained in these clinical pastoral care methods are able to take advanced units and specialize in general as well as specialized pastoral care ministry. It is typical for many hospitals to seek chaplains who have successfully completed four or more clinical pastoral care units. Clinical pastoral care chaplains can be ordained, religious, or laypersons, and are normally endorsed for hospital ministry by their faith tradition. Their basic training usually consists of religious studies, and perhaps a masters degree from a theological school. However, their defining criteria for ministry is successful completion of several supervised clinical pastoral ministry experiences. This competency is attested by their membership in a clinical pastoral organization such as the American Association of Clinical Pastoral Educators, and by their ability to function at an advanced clinical level.

Pastoral Care Educators

Pastoral care educators are those who have advanced clinical pastoral education training, and have completed supervisory training levels to become supervisors of clinical pastoral education departments. Their training level is the same as clinical pastoral care chaplains, but carries an added focus on the supervision and running of an accredited clinical pastoral education program in a hospital facility. As with the clinical pastoral care chaplain, educators can be ordained, religious, or laypersons, and usually have a masters degree in religious or theological studies. It is the tradition once a chaplain becomes a pastoral care educator, for him or her to stop or limit the provision of direct pastoral care and shift fairly extensively to the training of students. Frequently, the educator performs much of his or her clinical work indirectly through the supervision of students.

Pastoral Care Students

The final category in the clinical pastoral education tradition is that of "student." Students are mentioned because it is common to find them delivering pastoral care services directly to patients in hospitals, where such education programs exist. In fact, this is one of the benefits hospitals receive from participating in clinical pastoral education programs. Many students attend theological school and work on initial competencies appropriate to nonordained persons in the midst of masters level training while also working at the hospital. Their levels and capacities may change as their training progresses. In some cases, students move through the clinical training program with the sole intention of becoming educators and/or chaplains. Even more frequently, students are taking one clinical unit as required for ordination. The defining criteria, for students, is that they are engaged in a training program and are at the hospital to learn how to perform hospital visitation, specialized pastoral care, and/or chaplaincy.

Clinical Pastoral Counseling

The second type of clinical education in the category of newer traditions in hospital ministry, is that of clinical pastoral counseling. Pastoral counseling is an essential service that occurs in most hospital settings. It has become more recognized as clinical pastoral counseling has begun to be accepted as a competent therapy in the context of other disciplines such as clinical psychology, marriage and family therapy, Jungian analysis, and behavior therapy. Technically speaking, counseling has been a sound component of psychiatric hospital ministries for many years. However, today's clinically trained pastoral therapists are a welcome component in many hospital settings.

Clinical Pastoral Chaplains

Clinical pastoral chaplains who are trained in the field of pastoral counseling are able to provide crisis, brief, and longer term counseling services. These services may consist of individual, family, and group therapies, and may also be provided for staff, though usually on a brief basis, with referral services used frequently. Chaplains with counseling backgrounds may be more intimately involved with treatment teams, may provide intensive spiritual counseling as a component of therapy, and may provide supportive as well as primary therapy services. As chaplains, these individuals are likely to also be engaged in other pastoral care and administrative functions of a pastoral care chaplain. They may in some cases be members of accredited clinical pastoral care organizations as well as clinical pastoral counseling organizations. The hospital benefits from chaplains trained in both fields.

Pastoral Care Specialists

Pastoral care specialist is a new term for clergy who have advanced supervised experiences and who specialize in counseling within a parish and/or as chaplains. This field recognizes the growing need for counseling assessment, diagnosis, brief, and crisis therapies, and the growing need for more sophisticated referral resources. The defining criteria in this category include ordination and advanced supervision in counseling on common issues such as crisis intervention, grief and loss, divorce recovery, pastoral diagnosis, and making referrals.

Pastoral Counselors and Pastoral Psychotherapists

Pastoral counselors and pastoral psychotherapists in hospital ministry are those who focus on counseling and therapeutic services. This focus may be to the exclusion of other pastoral care functions or as part of their total ministry. These individuals are usually licensed or certified by state boards and certified by a counseling organization such as the American Association of Pastoral Counselors. They specialize in holistic treatment and in the expertise of having been trained in a variety of therapeutic schools as well as in the spiritual components of illness and health.

Pastoral Counseling Educators

A pastoral counseling educator's focus is on the supervision of students in pastoral counseling or other professional therapeutic fields that have a holistic focus. The pastoral counseling educator is usually a Diplomate in the American Association of Pastoral Counselors. Unless there are numerous students in a clinical program, the pastoral counseling educator engaged in full-time hospital ministry does not need to set aside as much time to direct the program as does a clinical pastoral care educator. The pastoral counselor educator may indeed have only one student being supervised at a given time. The size of the program, therefore, is quite flexible.

Counseling Interns and Residents

The nature of an internship or residency in pastoral counseling, or any related holistic counseling field, is such that students are not expected to devote as many hours to patients as pastoral care students would. They may, in fact, have anywhere from one to four patients/clients and lead one or two groups. They may receive didactic material in an academic setting or as part of the hospital's training program. Often they are expected to be working on graduate or postgraduate programs and come into hospital ministry and pastoral counseling at this advanced level.

RECENT DIRECTIONS

Postmodern Spirituality and Other Spiritual Care Ministry

A third area of hospital ministry (see Table 1.4) that is fairly recent in its growth is that of spiritual care coordinator. Spiritual care and spiritual care departments are sometimes chosen by hospitals rather than more traditional pastoral care and pastoral services departments. Some of the impetus for this growth and rise in interest is found in the social movement away from Jewish and Christian traditions and the increased religious plurality and diversity of our nation. In some cases, there is a decidedly intentional trend to separate spiritual care departments from identified faith traditions or traditionally trained chaplains and clergy.

Example

A community hospital struggled for years over the provision of services for hospitalized persons who were not active members in local congregations and therefore did not receive services from area clergy. Influential community leaders felt there should be a distinction between pastoral care (with its presumed religious connections) and spiritual care. The compromise for this hospital consisted of hiring a spiritual care coordinator who was an employee of the hospital who was working toward a degree in another helping profession.

Spiritual Care Chaplains and Coordinators

Spiritual care chaplains and coordinators may or may not be ordained. They may or may not have theological or religious studies in their backgrounds, and may have varied training experiences. These persons tend to use less language from Jewish and/or Christian religions and more from new age spiritualities, private beliefs, and popular spiritual experiences. They may have become chaplains and coordinators by moving from other disciplines such as social services and nursing.

Persons with Spiritual Care Focus

Persons with a spiritual care focus are usually individuals from other disciplines who work holistically with patients. They may have had formal spiritual care courses, or they may have been self-taught and thus conduct their work based on their own convictions. Frequently they accept the reality of mind, body, and spirit, and view this as part of health and healing. They may be connected to faith traditions and are certainly involved in helping patients connect spiritually as well as in other ways.

CHALLENGES AND CHANGES IN THE FIELD

As with any other health care discipline, hospital ministry seems to change by the minute. Some of these changes are driven by the changing needs of the patients and their families. Other changes are driven by the sources and nature of funding for services offered. Many changes are due to the evolution of health care and spiritual experiences and practices. The multiple contexts of hospital ministry make for changing factors, expectations, and practices. These changes bring questions, concerns, and challenges with them that must be addressed.

Who is competent to do what work?

The word "competency" is not a word typically found in the training of clergy and spiritual caregivers, nor in religious or spiritual care organizations. Yet the question of competency prevails in today's hospital setting. This question seeks to address specific categories of training and the skills required to deliver specified services. Health care competencies are usually constructed in a behavioral format. They are designed to be demonstrable to trained and untrained observers alike.

Earlier descriptions of hospital ministries and Tables 1.1 through 1.4 illustrate that at least thirteen categories of professionals are engaged in hospital ministry, and each category is based on a presumed set of competencies or skills. This proliferation of categories is significant since for many years hospital ministry consisted of one category: the community pastor, priest, rabbi or person from a religious order. The complex and growing diversification within the profession brings to the forefront the need for even more intense scrutiny over who is competent to provide which service.

The complexity of defining criteria, training, services, and customers may lead one to conclude that in order to meet this challenge, the diversity and skill base of current chaplains would have to increase. While this is quite feasible, increasing the number of chaplains to provide for greater diversity of services may be difficult in times when the rest of health care is downsizing and strictly managing care resources. Furthermore, in the next decade, formulations of explicit competencies for hospital ministry providers will only increase. So, the urgency remains for us to develop our own competencies, and to do so in conversation and consultation with others in the health care field.

Who is the customer in hospital ministry, and what is the customer's role?

As with all hospitals and disciplines, the question of "who is the customer" is of paramount importance, as is the practice of providing excellent customer service. Once thought to be a given, the ability to provide excellent customer service is now understood to be a significant factor in the choices patients make about which hospitals to use. Even those who are involuntarily hospitalized have the option to decline services that they dislike, that they feel do not meet their needs, or that are not conducted according to their wishes.

In the field of hospital ministry, chaplains serve many customers: patients, families, friends, and significant others. While serving the needs of these people, chaplains must also relate to hospital policies and procedures. They must recognize the varying needs of other internal and external customers such as churches, the community, managed care organizations, treatment teams, and legal interests. In addition, chaplains often feel a responsibility to God or a higher power, and to their calling. All customers, people, and processes gain the chaplain's attention.

It is no longer possible to claim that the chaplain's responsibility is solely to the patient. The use of the term "customer" changes the services provided and challenges previous notions of "doing for persons." Instead, today's focus is on increased partnership, collaboration, and empowerment. During the next decade the question of customer service will become even more crucial. Chaplains, in their primary role of meeting patient/family and staff needs are in a good position to provide leadership in this area.

How will positions be filled when there is a scarcity of personnel in some faith traditions?

The availability of trained personnel for hospital ministry is changing in a number of faith traditions. This is particularly true of ordained clergy. The number and average age of people in the process of training for ministry has changed dramatically in the past thirty to forty years. At this time, the majority of those in training for ministry are over age forty-five. In addition, it has been observed that a large percentage of clergy will reach retirement age within the next ten years. These changes, coupled with the closing, downsizing, and restructuring of many hospitals and departments, including hospital ministry departments, point to a potential scarcity of full-time hospital chaplains.

Example

There is a scarcity of Roman Catholic priests in New Hampshire. The Church struggles to find enough clergy for local churches and specialized ministries such as prisons, nursing homes, and hospitals. This situation is difficult for most hospitals in the state. Still, tradition has called for priests to be engaged in this type of ministry.

New Hampshire Hospital, an acute psychiatric facility, had a full-time Catholic chaplain for at least 150 years. No longer is this true. Since approximately 50 percent of its patients are of a Catholic background, it has been sorely taxed to provide the priestly services their patients desire. Currently, the hospital receives brief and limited services from a Eucharistic minister. They are quite grateful for these services.

A two-pronged approach to the scarcity of personnel is certainly possible, and it has been successfully used by pastoral care departments. Currently, chaplains must be available to all patients, families, and staff, regardless of faith tradition or belief. This works reasonably well and increases the skills of all chaplains. However, it requires intensive training for patients, family, and staff. In some situations, in fact, staff are resistant to accepting a "chaplain of all faiths," especially if the chaplain is not a priest. Continuous training as to the philosophy, mission, and changes in chaplaincy services is essential.

The availability of chaplains from traditional church groupings—Protestant, Catholic, and Jewish—is challenging, even in general hospitals run by churches and religious orders. For example, at Catholic Medical Center in Manchester, New Hampshire, there used to be six chaplains on staff. Now there are only two—a sister and a former member of a religious order. These chaplains provide services for persons of all faith traditions.

The second approach to the scarcity of personnel in some faith traditions is to build up the services of consults. Consults are trained and willing to provide services on either a voluntary or paid basis. However, changes in availability of such consults, and the willingness of hospitals to pay for these types of services, make this a more challenging approach.

How will we seriously address the ever-widening split between religious traditions, pastoral care, and spiritual care?

In a sense, there has always been a careful balancing and occasional territorial struggle among Protestant, Catholic, and Jewish chaplains. However, these balancing endeavors remain within the Judeo-Christian heritage that has represented the majority of American chaplains and patient/consumers. A balance has always been maintained by having "one of each" present, based on the location and prevalence of Jewish and Christian faith groups in a given community.

Currently, a growing plurality of religious and nonreligious beliefs has led to increased diversity of spiritual connections and needs. This plurality of beliefs is also influenced by the instant availability of a large number of world religions to just about every American. We are no longer, strictly speaking, a Christian country. Rather, we are now very much a part of the world global village, and are technologically connected to spiritual resources that would never have even been conceived of twenty years ago.

Example

In November 2000, an Internet search for "new age beliefs" brought 98,577 entries. On the same day, in the same hospital setting, a meeting was held about a joint endeavor called "Winter Connections." The endeavor was to be an educational and social opportunity for customers of the hospital to get together and build positive connections. A member of the Wellness Committee suggested that there be a Reike booth and a labyrinth. She was surprised to hear that these two practices had religious roots and came from traceable Christian and Eastern belief systems. The group glossed over the notion in silence. After a while, it was decided that a yoga demonstration was a good idea. Again, there was no thought of this being a spiritual practice. Five minutes after that, a committee member's response to a suggestion about having a customer service Santa was, "As long as there is no religion involved."

In many cases, religion and religious congregations have been placed in defensive positions. Actually, the tables have been turned and it may be pastoral care's turn to be challenged by other spiritual care individuals and organizations. However, many chaplains believe that attempts must be made to bring inclusivity to hospital ministry and demonstrate respect for all beliefs and traditions.

The reverse phenomenon of excluding traditional Jewish and Christian beliefs does not necessarily lead to meeting the needs of the majority of patients/consumers in some hospitals. The challenge, when addressing this ever-widening split, is to maintain all that is currently good about hospital ministry while moving into the future. This will happen through careful planning and assessment of patient needs. This approach appears to be a more creative path through a challenging situation.

Should students and interns be used to fulfill the functions of trained chaplains?

For a number of years, the trend of using students to meet the pastoral and spiritual care needs of patients has continued. Often, this approach fits well within the central focus of clinical pastoral education, in which students gain clinical pastoral care experience by providing services to patients and their families. However, these student-services are designed to be educational and thus provide a learning experience for the student. The issue is further complicated by hiring an insufficient number of trained chaplains, leaving the department to rely on a chaplain supervisor, who spends most of his or her time conducting the student-training program.

While it is true that students provide services that can be profoundly helpful, it is not true that these services meet the competencies required and expected of qualified chaplains. The challenge to hospitals and to hospital ministry is to view this as an issue of both funding and competency. Also, the challenge is one of use and possible abuse of students, whose primary function is learning, coupled with the consequent inadequate staffing of departments. The current situation has become somewhat of a tradition, and changes can only be introduced after looking at the broadest picture of hospital ministry possible, and noting the professional skills, functions, and professional personnel needed to fulfill the quality of services needed in this field.

How do we address the growing need for pastoral counseling and pastoral care specialists in hospital ministry?

Early in the twentieth century, when clinical pastoral education and clinical pastoral counseling were being developed, there was quite an overlap of hospital ministry services. Pastoral care programs focused on training ministers and persons in religious orders, most of whom were working on Master of Divinity degrees. Those interested in providing deeper and longer therapy services became credentialed in pastoral counseling, and many started providing services using church office space, counseling service centers, and private or group practices.

In recent years, clinical pastoral education organizations have made efforts to claim and vacate hospital ministry and clinical pastoral counseling, office space in hospitals. Although clinical pastoral education prepares chaplains for many functions within a pastoral care department, an increased need exists for advanced pastoral counseling in both general and specialty hospital settings. These endeavors may range from brief counseling services to long-term therapy.

There are three issues here. The first concerns services needed and how to best formulate and format these services from the patient/consumer perspective. The second issue has to do with competencies required to meet each service, and the third issue deals with providing integrative spiritual health care services rather than continuing the practice of "single focus" ministry.

How does our discipline address leadership, organizational and provider skills, and outcomes-based services required of chaplains as employees in "state-of-the art" health care settings?

Admittedly, most chaplains resist objectifying spiritual care services. To a certain degree, this resistance exists in other therapeutic disciplines as well. However, as chaplains, we have grown quite accustomed to the world of mystery. In fact, we embrace it rather openly as part our understanding of human limitations and the endless and ever-expanding work of the spirit. While some focus on the work of human hands, we focus on understanding that which may not be understandable.

As chaplains, we also work in a world dominated by scientific data and business acumen. In this world, data, outcomes, and skills take precedence over mysteries of the spirit. Ideas that can be demonstrated to work are kept, and those that do not are reviewed, improved, and/or changed.

This worldview and approach to health care leads to another challenge facing today's hospital ministry: how to incorporate the language and format of the hospital and retain the language and format of the ministry. The Apostle Paul would surely appreciate this dilemma. Well do those of us in the field of hospital ministry remember Paul's statement in Romans 12:2, "Do not be conformed to this world: but be transformed by the renewal of your mind, that you may prove what is the will of God, what is good and acceptable and perfect" (RSV). For many chaplains who come from a Christian background, these words constitute "marching orders" for how we conduct ourselves in the world outside the church's door.

However, most chaplains also need to engage in the activities of a "state of the art" hospital, which includes learning about surveys and accreditation, as well as identifying skills unique to us and how we know when services are adequately provided. At the same time we must be able to demonstrate our ministry in ways that are valuable. For this, we must learn to do a better job in teaching colleagues and consumers our language and desired outcomes. So, too, we must remain steadfast in our determination and call to embrace the movement of the spirit and the mystery of our God/Higher Power. We must do all of this as partners who have mutual goals at the heart of our purpose and mission in ministry. That is the challenge!

What is the role of local churches, synagogues, parishes, and parish clergy, and what could those roles be in the future?

Many hospitals in the United States do not have professional chaplains on staff. Numerous hospitals have part-time chaplains and/or situations where there is a need to rely heavily on the services of community churches and congregations for services within the hospital. For those hospitals with no professional chaplains or hospital ministry departments, there may not be training requirements, job descriptions, or comprehensive ways to discern the quantity or quality of spiritual care services. In many of these cases there are no services for patients who do not identify themselves with a specific congregation. To their credit, some of these hospitals rely heavily on the use and availability of volunteers.

At the same time, the rise of professional hospital ministries and chaplains has brought an increase in the quality of services and personnel in hospitals. However, hospital ministry has developed in much the same manner that local highway systems are maintained and repaired. When new traditions are added, they often are built right over the old, covering up both the good and the not so good aspects equally, or conversely, they are filled on a case-by-case basis. Just as potholes are filled each spring in New England, so too are decisions about the provision of services to local hospitals often left to the interests or lack of interests of local clergy and the prevailing care climate of individual hospitals. In some cases, the increasing strength of chaplaincy within a hospital leads to the retreat of local clergy and the prevailing assumption that "all that is taken care of" by them.

What has yet to be addressed extensively is the further integration and future role of churches in hospital ministry. Often, discussion and further action is dependent upon the development of simultaneous processes within hospital ministries and churches. This requires energy, sustained commitment, and initiative on both parts. It also requires time and leadership.

IN SUMMARY

The challenges facing hospital ministry, chaplains, caregivers, the Church, hospitals, and patient/consumers are profound and stem from changing health care concepts, processes, and an increasing diversity of spiritual care needs and services. Taken one by one, these challenges are not prohibitive by their nature, nor are they prohibitive in the ways they can be addressed. However, each challenge or question must be faced and answered in ways that look to the growing and

Chapter 2

Understanding the Hospitalization Process and Patient Needs

Caregiving includes an empathic quest for understanding how an individual is experiencing life. (Lester, 1995, p. 105)

MARTHA'S EXPERIENCE

The health care service system can be described as active prior to birth and throughout one's lifetime. Take Martha's experiences, for example. Martha was born forty-two years ago in a northeastern hospital on the north end of the city. Her mother had excellent prenatal services while she was expecting Martha. In fact, Martha's mother had two doctors. One was a general practitioner who had served Martha's family for many years, and the other was a gynecologist who came to the hospital and assisted in Martha's delivery. The delivery went well, and mother and baby stayed in the hospital three days following the birth.

Throughout Martha's childhood, she had regular checkups with a pediatrician. Once, she fell down and cut her leg. The bleeding was so intense that she was taken to the hospital nearest her house and received emergency services. Martha received six stitches in her leg and directions for follow-up care at home. Later, she went to her doctor's office to have the stitches removed. When Martha turned eighteen she continued having regular checkups with their long-time family doctor, and began seeing a gynecologist when she was in college. At age twenty-four, Martha gave birth to a son and stayed in the hospital for two days postpartum. She received similar services at age twenty-six when she gave birth to another son. Martha began taking vitamins and supplements in her mid-thirties and paid special attention to exercise and heart-healthy eating.

During a routine checkup at age forty-two, Martha's gynecologist discovered a large growth near her ovaries, and she was sent for an ultrasound. The test showed that the growth was the size of an orange and was located on her left ovary. Martha was sent immediately for a blood test which came back negative for cancer.

After several conversations with her gynecologist, who was also a surgeon, surgery was scheduled within three weeks to remove the growth. Martha received instructions on pre-op procedures and education about the surgery and possible choices and outcomes. The doctor planned to remove the growth and the ovary, and look around for additional growths. During the operation, a test on the growth confirmed that it was benign and the doctor felt that there was no more work to be done.

Martha came out of recovery to find her husband waiting for her. The nurses were friendly, efficient, and attentive to some pain she began feeling on the second day. A couple of friends visited Martha, as did the hospital chaplain. She went home on the third day after her surgery. Her mother came into town to help. On the evening of the third day, Martha began her at-home recovery that was anticipated to last two to six weeks. She had a follow-up appointment with her gynecologist in three weeks. She returned to work part time. By the end of the fifth week she was back to work full time and said she felt fine.

THE HEALTH CARE SERVICE WHEEL

Martha's health care experiences were common and led to a positive view of the health care system and to increased confidence in the ability to receive quality care and timely services. The scope of services provided was well explained and she had ample opportunity to ask questions and to rely on her doctor, friends, and clergy for support during her times of concern and fear. In a matter of several weeks, Martha had health care services that covered the entire health care service wheel, indicated in Figure 2.1. She experienced several smooth transitions aided by an abundance of resources.

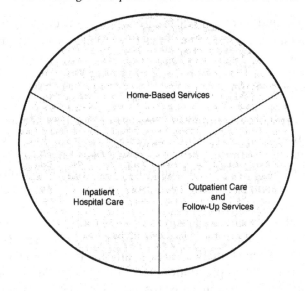

FIGURE 2.1. Health Care Service Wheel Continuum of Care

Briefly described, the health care service wheel is a continuum of care model based on the location of where health care services are provided. When these services are seen as connective and collaborative, patients, family, and professionals experience a sense of emotional trust and well-being even though the health care issue may be intense and constitute a difficult and painful experience. When there are obstacles in the delivery and quality of services at any point on the service wheel, or between points, stress occurs. This stress may lead to a variety of negative consequences for all involved.

Services are provided at each location on the health care service wheel. Smooth connections between services are ideal; however, since this is not always the case and services vary in each location, there are always challenges that arise in the system. Along with these challenges there are specific expectations for transitions along the service continuum. Understanding this service model and the current philosophy of health care is crucial for parish pastors, lay leaders, hospital clergy, and spiritual care providers. Also essential to hospital and parish ministry is the realization that there is often confusion about the health care continuum and the health care services wheel.

Better understanding of the health care system can help spiritual caregivers understand, relate, and advocate the concerns of patients, staff, and families.

Home-Based Health Care

The underpinnings of quality home-based health care are education and prevention. Abundant resources are available to encourage lifestyle changes with the intention of increasing an individual's capacity to provide good self-care and therefore increase personal wellness. These educational and preventative efforts have brought about a diversity in health care options.

Many of these health care strategies are solidly based on research findings. For example, the use of vitamins, exercise, low-fat diets, and stress reduction strategies are a common part of home treatment for wellness and illness prevention. Holistic strategies that seek to integrate mind, body, and spirit are also available. These strategies may include meditation, prayer, devotional reading, and other spiritual care practices.

However, home-based health care can be confusing. This confusion can add to the burden consumers sometimes feel about managing their health at home. For example, the abundance of information and choices available can be overwhelming, and professional opinions can vary. In addition, the high cost of health care can limit its accessibility to those with limited funds. These factors have led some to contend with health care situations that require a different treatment than is available or can be afforded. Patients have had to be more aware of coverage issues and more assertive in getting the services they want or need.

Inpatient Hospital Care

Hospital care has always been set aside for medical and mental conditions that cannot be treated while the consumer remains at home. With the exception of individuals with health care needs that are extensive and longer term, the majority of people spend only a brief amount time in inpatient hospital settings. For these patients who are reasonably healthy throughout their lifespan, such services account for a tiny portion of their total health care needs. These brief services are called acute care services. When people are hospitalized, once they have been treated and their condition has stabilized they are discharged. Most people experience their health care services under the home-based continuum of care.

At the other extreme are individuals who require extensive inpatient services due to complicated and sometimes chronic health problems. In these cases of intense, lengthy hospitalization, there are also increased financial, supportive, and therapeutic needs. Such services may be carried out in acute care facilities, long-term units, or long-term hospital settings. Financial complications, as well as availability and choice of services, have added to the burden for both service providers and patient/consumers who need such extended and intensive services.

Example

Nellie was in her eighties when she was hospitalized for hip replacement surgery at a general hospital. Her hospitalization took place in the mid-1980s, prior to managed care. The replacement was successful and Nellie was able to sit up and move a little bit. She had been in the hospital for over six weeks and was medically stable, although somewhat frail. Because Nellie could not return to her own home, and because it was not easy to find the kind of assistance she needed, Nellie remained in the hospital in kind of a step-down unit. Under some circumstances, Nellie would have received only the surgery followed by a fairly speedy return home. However, her age and her health care needs meant that she needed services not yet in place and that required time to arrange. The health care service system was doing its best to help meet Nellie's needs. It just was not able to move fast enough and Nellie's hospitalization was lengthy.

Outpatient Care and Follow-Up Services

Today patients are leaving the hospital much earlier than would have been imagined ten to fifteen years ago. Women who give birth in hospitals often must fight to remain in the hospital two days. A three-day stay in the hospital is considered lengthy, and two days is about average for general hospitals. Acute psychiatric patients stay an average of about twelve days. Naturally, this means that health care continues after the patient returns home from the hospital.

Extended services, where inpatient resources are still needed, occasionally take place at specialty hospitals such as rehabilitation centers. If inpatient services are deemed unnecessary, follow-up care may happen through visits back to the hospital. When such is the case, these services are called outpatient services.

Wrap-Around or Seamless Services

Today's hospital is but one component among a variety of health care resources available. A proliferation of services has led to increased efforts to provide quality services regardless of where an individual is on the service wheel. Furthermore, not only are patient's needs expected to be met within each category of the wheel, but these expectations carry from one service model to the other as a person progresses from one service to another and vice-versa. This means that interconnection and collaboration are very important.

CHANGES IN HOSPITALIZATION AND CARE

Length of Stay

In general hospitals, most patients are admitted and released within one or two days. Patients who stay three or more days view their hospitalization with even greater concern. Even with the changes in length of stay, there continues to be a number of consumers whose illnesses call for hospital stays of three days or more. However, many treatment functions that used to be part of inpatient hospital services are now considered outpatient services and are done at home, in doctor's offices, as day patients, or in rehabilitation hospitals.

The same can be said for psychiatric services. At New Hampshire Hospital, a tertiary acute care psychiatric facility, one-third of admitted patients stay one to three days. Another one-third may stay up to ten days while one-third of patients stay more than ten days. The average length of stay in this facility is twelve days. These figures are amazing when compared to the past. When patients were sent to this type of hospital, they were sometimes there for the rest of their lives!

In some cases, the differences in length of hospitalization can be attributed to treatment interventions currently available that were not available twenty, thirty, or fifty years ago. In other cases, the length of hospitalization has changed due to increased availability of services for outpatient and follow-up care. It may also be true that patients actually prefer to heal in their own home setting.

Focus of Treatment

Not only has the average length of hospital stay changed dramatically, so has the focus of treatment. The focus today is on rapid intervention and rapid stabilization, a point at which community care services can be effectively utilized. The belief that one goes to a hospital to be cured of a disease is no longer operative in the health care field, even though patients, family, and friends may still think so. For example, a person does not go to the hospital to be cured of cancer or heart disease. Rather, they go to obtain rapid interventions that help an acute episode of cancer growth or heart malfunction. This, too, in a way, is only an initial part of treatment. The rest occurs outside hospital or on an outpatient basis.

Likewise, a person does not go to a psychiatric hospital to be cured of bipolar disorder. Rather, a person goes to such a hospital to help stablize symptoms through medication and other hospital-based services. Rapid interventions are made in instances such as this so the patient may remain alive, be safe, and in some cases be forced to follow a medical regimen that might not make sense to a person in the throws of a major mental illness episode.

Voluntary Admissions

Most admissions to hospitals are voluntary. This means that the consumer decides to go to the hospital. In the case of children, parents and/or guardians often make the decision. Most noncrisis admissions are scheduled ahead of time, and in some cases, patients are admitted for what is termed elective surgery. All of these types of admissions are based on the willingness, desire, or acceptance of the individual to go to a hospital and receive recommended treatment. Persons who enter hospitals voluntarily are assumed to have given consent to treatment and to be capable or competent of giving this consent. In general, voluntary patients do not resist treatment although do make choices concerning the treatment they receive.

Involuntary Admissions

Some persons do not choose to be admitted to a general or specialty hospital. This can be the case for those who have or may be diagnosed with a psychiatric illness. In tertiary care psychiatric facilities and designated psychiatric receiving settings, a person may be admitted against his or her wishes. A doctor, community mental health assessment team, and several witnesses can be brought together and have a person committed involuntarily for up to three days. At the end of three days the person must have a legal court hearing to determine whether the original cause for emergency hospitalization was just, and whether the person should be confined for treatment for an additional time. If no cause is found, the person may leave the hospital. If probable cause is found to keep the patient, the person remains in the facility and is encouraged to receive treatment for an additional seven days.

In emergency cases, treatment may be temporary in order to keep the individual safe. After ten days, the hospital treatment team can either ask the court to have the patient committed to the hospital for a longer time, or indicate that the patient is medically stable enough to leave. If the patient needs further treatment, and does not willingly participate in such treatment, then a treatment team may seek a guardian for the patient until such time as the patient is deemed competent to make treatment decisions.

William's Experience

William was in his middle twenties when he found himself admitted to a tertiary care psychiatric facility. His admission meant that he could not be cared for in his home and community (known as primary care), nor could he be cared for in a psychiatric unit within a general hospital (secondary care). The reason he was admitted to a tertiary care psychiatric facility was because he wanted to die and had homicidal thoughts about another individual in the community. William was a bright young man who had no previous history of hospitalization, but acknowledged during his course of treatment that he had struggled with depression much of his young life. It was difficult for William and his team to know how much of his depression was due to developmental issues and trauma from his childhood, and how much was due to situational depression stemming from a combination of physical injury, job loss, and current family problems.

William was successful at his job until his injury. He had tried to be a good parent and struggled in his marriage. William had no identified spiritual beliefs but had a great interest in attending groups in which spirituality was part of the therapy. He had no place to go, and in fact, was afraid of leaving the hospital. He did not consider himself well enough to leave.

WHAT DO PATIENTS WANT?

One Hospital's Story

Mercy Hospital is known as a state-of-the art hospital. This means that it is accredited according to strict standards and provides outstanding services compared to similar hospitals throughout the United States. The hospital has been providing services for almost 160 years and has seen many changes. Early in the 1990s the hospital hired a consultant to train high-level and middle managers in ways of quality improvement such as is now commonly found in the corporate business world. There really wasn't much resistance to this training or to the institution of a quality improvement council. In fact, many improvement teams came and went, and in general, the hospital seemed to go from really good to even better!

Seven years later the quality council, consisting solely of the hospital's executive committee plus three highly placed manager/consultants, began to wonder about the larger issue of improving customer service. This coupled with a natural desire to be an outstanding health care facility led to the formation of a customer service improvement team. They found that process-wise, everything looked good. Thus, neither the hospital nor the team was able to move quickly on anything new. Three years and a consultant later, a comprehensive plan was sent to the quality council and then to the executive committee. Here's why:

Along the way, a staff survey had been conducted by the customer service team. A focus group provided staff feedback to the team. In a totally unrelated survey, staff were asked to provide feedback about their work and experience at the hospital. When the consultant came on board, a third survey went out to all staff. This was followed up by focus groups. Everyone on the team felt that they had gained valuable information and feedback from one rather important set of customers—hospital staff.

In the first month after its formation the customer service review committee, under the direction and accountability of the executive committee, began to formulate its vision and mission regarding customer service at Mercy. The committee wondered, in particular, how it would get individuals and departments to assess their customer service, versus the needs and expectations of their customers. They turned rather quickly to an exercise known as a service matrix.

The committee was quite pleased to find that with a bit of work they could figure out how to fill in this matrix. Furthermore, they felt they could complete the section concerning staff needs, as they had already completed surveys and focus group information for these sets. Since Mercy had always considered the patient to be the first and primary customer, filling out the key expectations of patients seemed to be equally easy at first glance.

The committee gathered around the large administrative table after lunch on a late spring day. Everyone was ready to get to the task at hand. A person who had worked on the project from the beginning started with a question: "How do we know, other than from hearsay, experience, or anecdotal information, what patients at Mercy really want and expect from us?"

There was silence. The silence was followed by the response, "How about the patient satisfaction survey?" Most people on the committee were aware of the survey and reviewed it in their minds. They realized immediately that members of the executive committee had designed the survey from a list of areas and services that they thought were important to patients. A small percentage of patients filled out these surveys. Nowhere on the survey was there a space for patients to list their expectations, needs, and priorities!

RESEARCH ON WHAT PATIENTS WANT

The best patient surveys available are based on the combined wisdom of consumers and health care providers, and on solid data gained through quality research. With these caveats in mind, humility demands that we realize that the wishes, expectations, and needs of patients are an essential part of health care delivery and essential to recovery. Second, although patients may be highly satisfied with surveyed services, they may be deeply dissatisfied about other areas that are important to them as individuals. A patient can fill out a satisfaction survey and still have essential needs that may not have been met.

For these reasons a brief review of patients needs, represented in recent research, is presented throughout the rest of this chapter. This review is not intended to be exhaustive. Rather, it provides examples, ideas, and brief exposure to the challenging task of asking the essential question, "What do patients need, want, and expect?"

It is helpful to be exposed firsthand to the answers patients have given, and to hear about the priorities they set for health care services. Because the needs of hospitalized persons are multiple and complex, and because their voices need to be heard, the responses are included in patients' own words. In most cases, the top preferences from specific research are the ones included.

Attributes Desired When Choosing a Family Physician

- Takes your concerns seriously
- Explains results and options clearly
- Spends time with you; is not hurried
- Is easy to confide in
- Listens without interrupting (Engstrom and Madlon-Kay, 1998, p. 24)

General Practice Wishes

- Enough time during consultation
- Quick services in case of emergencies
- Confidentiality of information
- Tell patients all they want to know
- Make patients feel free to talk about their problems (Groll et al., 1999, p. 7)

When Breaking Bad News About Cancer

- A private, quiet, comfortable setting without interruptions
- Use of simple and direct language
- Talk to patient in person before discussing with family
- Be truthful
- Convey hope (Kim and Alvi, 1999, pp. 1066-1067)

What Psychiatric Patients Want Most

- Clarification—help putting feelings, thoughts, behaviors into perspective or to help when making a decision
- Psychological expertise—explanations as to why patients think, feel, or act in the ways they do
- Psychodynamic insight—talk about roots of their problems with hopes that understanding will lead to change
- Desire to make decisions for themselves (Noble, Douglass, and Newman, 1999, p. 324)

Preferences of Elders Regarding Life-Sustaining Treatment

- Order less LST for physical and mental impairment and more for metastatic cancer
- Use CPR more and artificial feeding less
- Prefer non-invasive interventions
- Prefer quality of life rather than length of life (Carmel, 1999, pp. 1405-1406)

Questions Asked When a Person Has Prostate Cancer

- Options?
- If not treat will I die?
- If delay treatment what are chances of being cured?
- If not treat how fast will cancer spread?
- If not treat what parts of body could be affected? (Feldman-Stewart et al., 2000, p. 11)

Should Physicians Ask About Spiritual/Religious Beliefs
if Patient Gravely Ill?

- Yes if the patient is gravely ill (Ehman et al., 1999, p. 1803)

*Spiritual Needs and Wishes of Psychiatrically
Ill Persons*

- Want pastor/rabbi/spiritual advisor to not abandon them
- Ask person about religious/spiritual preference
- Contact person mentioned
- Focus on comfort, companionship, conversation, and consolation (Moller, 1999, pp. 8-10)

Summary of Research Regarding Patients' Wishes and Needs

Looking at this brief literature search we can make some assumptions about what patients want from health care professionals.

Patients want health care professionals to:

- Spend time with them
- Listen
- Take their concerns seriously
- Keep confidentiality
- Use simple and direct language
- Explain diagnosis, results, causes, and treatment options
- Be truthful
- Convey hope
- Give information needed
- Help but let them make their own decisions
- Focus on quality of life not length
- Request preferences for noninvasive interventions
- Ask about spiritual/religious beliefs or preferences if gravely ill
- Talk to patient before family

Patients want clergy to:

- Ask about spiritual/religious beliefs and preferences
- Focus on comfort, companionship, conversation, and consultation

A General Hospital Determines Patients' Needs

Once an exhaustive literature search of current research concerning patient wishes and needs has been conducted it is possible to make generalizations. These generalizations can be the basis of individualized surveys. To be sure, there is great value in conducting one's own opportunities for feedback. In fact, Beverly Hospital in Beverly, Massachusetts, went a step further and hired a consultant to help them answer the following two questions: "What do patients and families really want," and "what do patients say?" Following is what Beverly Hospital found in 1999 (Stanley, 2000).

What Patients and Families Really Wanted

- Emotional support
- Professional, competent care providers
- Introduction of each team member
- Meals at their discretion
- Prompt attention
- Lights answered ASAP
- Clean rooms
- Organized discharge care

What Patients Said

Patients at Beverly Hospital indicated that they wanted:

- To be able to understand the answers to their questions
- To have test results explained in a way they could understand
- To be able to completely discuss their anxieties and fears
- To have families/friends more involved in discharge education
- To have more information about medication side effects at home
- To know when normal activity can resume

These findings seem to articulate patients' feelings that improvement in these areas would bring about better care for themselves and others. The hospital agreed and instituted what it calls "Patients First," a program of training hospital staff to better meet the needs of patients, and their families and friends.

WHAT PATIENTS WANT IN THE AREA
OF SPIRITUAL CARE

There are numerous ways to determine what patients want in the area of spiritual care. The next section of this chapter will provide information about patients' wishes and concerns. The first example is based on patient responses to what are known as chaplain request forms. For those who wish to try this approach, a sample form is provided in Appendix B. The second example is based on information gathered during a patient focus group. Both of these examples come from patients hospitalized in a psychiatric facility. The third example comes from patient responses while visiting with chaplain interns in a general hospital. This information was gathered from intern progress notes and verbatims.

A Psychiatric Hospital Determines Spiritual Care Needs of Patients

The Use of Chaplain Request Forms

For the past twelve years, patients at New Hampshire Hospital in Concord have received a pastoral service brochure and a chaplain request form upon admission. The brochure contains descriptions of the department's vision, mission, personnel, and services. Patients who wish to request services are instructed to fill out the chaplain request form and leave it at the nursing station. Additional forms are available in each unit. Patients, family, visitors, and staff may also contact pastoral services by phone or through any one of the chaplains or other hospital staff.

The chaplain request form includes the following eight categories:

1. Initial visit
2. Worship information
3. Pastoral care visit
4. Counseling
5. Prayer
6. Sacrament/Rite
7. Literature/Bible
8. Family support

In an effort to determine the services most frequently requested by patients in the simplest way possible, volunteers were asked to tally recent requests on selected chaplain request forms. Responses written in the space marked "other" were also tallied. After tabulating a sample of 200 forms, it was possible to determine the most frequently requested services during a one-year period. This brief sampling of chaplain request forms did not include the large number of service requests that came to the department verbally and over the phone. Nevertheless, several interesting results were noted. (See data review of patient requests in Appendix C.)

Learning About Services Requested

The first thing that was learned as a result of this review was that some patients were aware of the pastoral services request form and used it. Questions of whether services should be added to the list and concerns about the clarity and understanding of certain services were raised. Most important, an insightful tool—the chaplain request form—was reviewed for its effectiveness as an instrument for identifying and improving services. Thus, the task of improving services was based on a better understanding of patient needs from *their* perspective. A summary of feedback from this review follows.

The Most Requested Services

The four most requested services of chaplains in this psychiatric hospital were:

1. Initial visit
2. Literature/Bible
3. Counseling
4. Prayer

Patients want to receive an initial visit by the chaplain. For some patients the first visit is of crucial importance. By combining the categories of initial visit and pastoral care visit, it becomes clear that "presence" is still the most desired intervention from chaplains. At the same time, not everyone wants a general visit. Some have other specific services that are of greater importance. However, any of these other services are also likely to include an initial visit from the chaplain as a secondary gain.

Some requests are specific. Some patients will request either a priest, minister, rabbi, or born-again chaplain. Since there are many patients who do not fill out forms, it is possible to assume that an initial visit from a chaplain might very well be positively received in some cases. Likewise, there are patients who do not wish services of any kind from the chaplain or other clergy and spiritual care providers. These situations are always determined on an individual basis or through other forms of communication. As a result, the chaplain request form provides information about service preferences for about one-sixth of the patient population in a given year.

Patients want to receive literature and/or the Bible. These requests are often for devotional and self-care material. Particularly desired during the selected sample period were booklets of prayers, King James Bibles, favored hymns, and daily devotional guides. There were also single requests for the Talmud and the Koran. Those who were unable to come to the chapel also requested care notes around themes of grief and loss, illnesses and recovery, self-care, and relationships.

Patients request counseling. At this hospital, pastoral counseling is a recognized therapy. Consequently there are numerous referrals from staff for brief and long term counseling by qualified chaplains. This counseling is done in consultation with the treatment team and relates to treatment goals. In this survey, it was confirmed that patients also had a strong preference for counseling from chaplains. This feedback affirmed a prior departmental decision to increase individual and group counseling efforts.

Patients request prayer. One-third of patients who requested services from the pastoral services department over a one-year period requested prayers. We believe that the verbal requests for prayers may be much higher than this percentage. In this hospital, prayers are believed to be an important part of recovery and spiritual health. At least half of prayer requests, written and verbal, involve an intercessory type of experience. This may be related to the fact that approximately one-half of the patients in this hospital come from a Roman Catholic background. Usually, when these prayers are requested, it is understood that they are to be said on the patient's behalf at a time other than with the patient. Those who do not have a Roman Catholic influence often expect a prayer to be said with them, and all appreciate being kept on a chaplain's prayer list. It is important to check individual preferences and practices in following up on prayer requests.

Unclear Services

The reason for the small number of requests for Sacraments/Rites is unclear. Only 22 percent of requests were for communion. The term "Sacrament/Rite" was originally used as a way of being open to Baptists, for example, who have ordinances rather than sacraments. "Sacraments/Rites" provided outside of Sunday services are less in demand. In hospitals where communion is provided daily, and in those where there are no Sunday services, there may be more patients receiving communion. In this case, more information needs to be gathered in order to understand whether this service accurately represents the wishes of patients, or whether the way it is worded on the request form is confusing.

Building New Services

Family support is a growing category of services requested. Several years ago the pastoral services department responded to a patient-family education improvement process and rethought services to families. Thus, "Family support" was added to the chaplain request form. For a few years there were almost no requests for family support services from patients through the use of this form, which is not to say that there weren't any requests for family support families and staff. However, during this last sampling, it was found that use of the request form for family support significantly increased by 15 percent. In the case of new categories such as this, changes must be noted over time.

Service Changes Made

After the sample of chaplain request forms were tallied, the chaplains reviewed requests made through other channels. This review was based on anecdotal information gained through day-to-day experience. Consequently several modifications were made to the original chaplain request form. Four new categories were added:

1. Communion (formerly Sacraments/Rites)
2. Holy Communion for Catholics (formerly Sacraments/Rites)
3. Cross/Rosary
4. Spiritual Care Resources

Adding communion choices. For most of the hospital's 158 years, there have been Protestant and Catholic chaplains, and therefore, worship and Mass on Sundays. Communion was always available upon request from these ordained clergy. However, patients were encouraged to attend worship or Mass. As times changed, priests were no longer available for Mass and in most cases no longer provided Holy Communion. The chaplain request form had not been adjusted to reflect these changes.

The availability of a Eucharistic minister once again brought the service of Holy Communion to Roman Catholics. This led to an opportunity to provide the categories for Communion and Holy Communion for Catholics. The change is much clearer than the previous category although there has been no apparent increase in requests for either form of Communion.

Adding a category for crosses and rosaries. For many years the pastoral services department has realized that a large number of patients request crosses and rosaries. However, there was no change undertaken to include these two items on a revised form. While just a handful of forms included written-in requests for these items during the sample period, it was determined that these items are likely to be as highly requested as prayers. It will be interesting to see how including these resources in the request form changes the nature and amount of requests in this area.

Adding the category of spiritual care resources. The terms "spiritual" and "spirituality" are increasingly popular terms. Patients who do not belonging to specific traditional churches are less likely to respond to some of the traditional services such as pastoral care, communion, Bibles, and crosses. As this number increases in the hospital setting, the need for a wider variety of spiritual care resources increases. After monitoring this new category for an extended period it will be possible to determine specific resources requested and decide whether adding more specific categories are needed.

A Sensitive Category Noted

No change was made to request form regarding escort to church. The only other type of written-in request in this sample was for an escort to church on Sundays. In a psychiatric facility, this is a complicated request resting on a delicate balance of determining factors such as patient safety, privileges, and staff availability.

Equally important is the pastoral care department's inability to provide an escort on a regular basis. By listing this service on a request form we would be suggesting a service that could not be delivered. Hence there was no change made here.

Request Forms Indicate Trends and Specify Patient Needs

Information from request forms and the knowledge of seasoned chaplains were both used to create changes in the services listed on revised request forms. Doing this on a regular basis ensures that one can keep in touch with the needs of the patients served. Sometimes keeping things simple, such as the way the request forms were tabulated, can be just as helpful. Also, using a tool already in place ensures a greater possibility of getting the job done. For those with no written data about the wishes and needs of patients, instituting a chaplain request form would be a possible place to begin.

The Use of Focus Groups

To Determine Barriers to Spiritual Care and Recovery

Focus groups can also be a helpful way to identify wishes and needs. Focus groups can consist of any mix of customers, consumers, and employees. However, many hospitals do not gather much information about patients' wishes and needs in this kind of less structured format. At New Hampshire Hospital, the department of pastoral services undertook such a project. The department had easy access to ongoing therapeutic group time through its established groups called "Conversations with the Chaplain," "Loss and Recovery," and "Spiritual Care and Recovery."

Over a period of two weeks, a portion of these weekly groups was set aside to talk about patient wishes and needs regarding spiritual and pastoral care. A brainstorming activity was conducted. During this time patients were asked to respond to the following questions:

- What are the barriers or obstacles to spiritual care and recovery?
- What do you want or need when you are facing these obstacles?

It quickly became evident that many participants really liked answering these questions. Some found it painful but still worthwhile. Others seemed to use the group discussion for immediate help in areas of concern to them. A number of patients continued the conversation in consequent sessions.

The patient-identified barriers to spiritual care and recovery are listed in Tables 2.1 and 2.2. The words used come directly from patients and represent their perceptions. The responses are primarily to the first question.

Answers to the question of barriers to spiritual care and recovery came quite quickly. However, the task of responding to wants or needs when facing the identified barrier became laborious for many patients. In some cases group leaders determined that the wishes and needs column was implied in the barrier description, and was a bit

TABLE 2.1. Barriers to Spiritual Care and Recovery

Internal Barriers	Wishes and Needs
Feel I am not good/I am unworthy	
Not know own story	
Not focus on own gifts	To know what gifts I have, if any
Not using gifts on self	
Not have strength to use self-help resources	
Concentration and processing information is difficult	To take my medication and have it work
Too spiritual/religious?	To know one way or the other
Not individualize spiritual care	
Competing needs	To be able to do what is most important
Lack of self-discipline to carry out practices	
Problems with authority when told what to do/not do—anger	To make my own decisions
Lack of commitment and integration	
Not focus on self	
Spirit/Body split	
Low/Loss of self-esteem	
Being too impressionable	
Fears	
Feelings of guilt	

TABLE 2.2. Barriers to Spiritual Care and Recovery

External Barriers	Wishes and Needs
Practice Problems	
Not doing the program or practices	To practice my beliefs daily
Unable to pray or read Bible	
Not going to church	
Trying to do too much	To do what I can do and set the rest aside
Not doing enough	
Too much religion	
Hard to understand, follow, practice what the Bible says	Help from others
Externalizing and proselytizing	
Theory can be impractical—hard to break down into practices	Someone to talk to who will be practical and easy to understand
People and Relationships	
Relying on others' thoughts, feelings, beliefs	To be confident in what I believe
External story not nice—not to know how to edit, keep/drop threads and carry others through on a daily basis	To recover and change my story about who I am
Other people's reactions	
No family support	To have family be supportive
Difficult dealing with people who don't believe—feel responsibility to teach word	To not feel so guilty about trying to save people
Experience persecution/resistance	
Hard to relate to church communities	A church I like

tedious for the patient to restate. In other cases, it seemed that some patients and peers in the group had limited thoughts about their wishes and needs due to limited insight surrounding the obstacle/barrier. In a few cases, the participants just could not focus on the discussion any longer.

What to Do with Information Gathered from Focus Groups

Focus groups are used when one wants to get a quick response. Information gathered from these focus groups can provide a quick "feel" for thoughts, feelings, and responses for the subject under consideration. In this sense, the focus group is like a quick temperature check. Information obtained can be useful in pointing to other information needed as well as to how to proceed with 'the next step in a given area. The greatest asset of focus groups is that they are relational and spontaneous. Information is gained that might never be gained in a survey or more structured process. However, the focus group is limited in that it is not necessarily all-encompassing nor can its contents be checked for statistical validity.

Once one has gathered information from a focus group, the information must be processed in some manner. The usual processing of this kind of information is to make a list of what is said and to categorize the remarks into usable groupings. Once groupings or themes are found, decisions can be made as to prioritizing the information and deciding perhaps, what to do next. One can get quite fancy and put information on flow charts or graphs. The most important outcome of this process is a sense of what is going on. In the example discussed earlier, we get a sense of our patients' wishes and needs using this method, and knowing this helps us deliver the best care possible.

Spiritual Care Needs of Patients in a General Hospital

What Patients Tell Interns About Their Wishes and Needs

A third way of gathering information about patients' wishes and needs is through the review of clinical pastoral education verbatim and process notes. In this next example, the process consisted of reviewing verbatim and process notes from 1,902 visits made by clinical pastoral education students in a general hospital setting during an extended unit of study that ended in the spring of 2000. This review consisted of looking for words and phrases that indicated the wishes of patients. Instances when the patient did not indicate or initiate a preference, and in those occasions when the chaplain intern initiated the subject, were omitted.

About health concerns. In this survey of verbatim and process, patients, generally speaking, told the chaplain interns that they wanted:

- To be discharged and to go home (although they often had some concerns about going home)
- To be pain free and to know what was causing their pain

- To be well (healed)
- To have clear diagnoses, and have results from tests as soon as possible, and have some general resolution to their health condition
- To sleep and be rested and not have some types of treatment
- To have professionals stop by, even if briefly

About family and friends. Patients spoke frequently about their families and of their separation from family members. A number of patients were lonely and wanted support from family members and friends. Often that support was experienced when a family member or friend came to the hospital for a visit. Parents were often quite clear that they missed their children and wanted the children to be able to visit with them in the hospital. Also, patients worried about family members who were also ill. Visiting families were often direct in their conversations with the chaplain interns regarding wishes and needs. On many occasions the chaplain interns found themselves providing pastoral care to patients through their families.

About feelings. Patients often expressed to chaplain interns expectations they had for themselves. Some of these expectations were difficult to manage and caused feelings of frustration during pastoral care visits. These feelings, expectations, and frustrations were frequently followed by the desire/need to:

- Refrain from crying
- Stay hopeful
- Experience comfort
- Celebrate being healed
- Not feel helpless
- Experience being cared about

About the future. Some patients told chaplains that they found illness and hospitalization provided opportunities for them to:

- Start over/begin a new life
- Reflect on what would be next in life
- Have another chance to live

What Patients Tell Interns About Their Needs/Wishes Regarding Services from Chaplains and Clergy

About prayer requests. When patients wanted visits from chaplains they primarily wanted someone to supportively listen to them. They were open to prayer, which was usually suggested by the chaplain interns. Of 1,902 visits only twenty-nine patients specifically asked for prayers, and thirteen specifically declined prayers when suggested by the intern. However, the chaplain interns indicated that they prayed with about 75 percent of patients and families visited.

About practices. Other practices that a very small number of patients requested were:

• A blessing
• Clergy from a specific faith group
• Communion
• Confession

About devotional aids. Only a handful of patients requested devotional aids. These persons either asked for a Bible, a New Testament, the Psalms, or a specific devotional booklet. One person requested a rosary.

About visits from the chaplain. From the verbatim and process notes it was unclear how many of the 1,902 patients who were visited actually requested the visit. The content of the notes, however, implied that there were many requests to see chaplains. Although chaplains regularly visited patients, only a few patients felt the need to ask directly for the chaplain to return. A handful of patients declined visits from the chaplain because of the timing of the chaplain's visit or because they did not want a visit. Many patients simply wanted someone to talk to while others did not. One person expressed the need for someone—anyone—to listen. Two others wanted to not feel so alone, and two additional patients indicated that they wanted to be saved from boredom. In sum, support and prayer appeared to be the most highly valued components of pastoral care visits based on responses of gratitude regarding chaplain's visits and the content recorded about the visit.

About chaplains touching them. One patient reached out to touch a chaplain, grabbing the chaplain's hand and declaring, "Help me, help me." This wish was not noted in other places so it is difficult to know, from the content of the review, what the patient's preferences are regarding touch.

About the chaplain. Some patients wanted to know the denomination of the chaplain intern. Frequently, the patient responded that denomination made no difference. Others were interested to know more about the role of the chaplain intern. Twice patients wanted to know what they could do for the chaplain. These persons felt ill at ease about what the chaplain wanted from them.

What Patients Tell Interns About Their Wishes and Needs from God

Significant portions of conversations with chaplain interns were about faith, spiritual issues, and beliefs. A small number of patients—twenty of the 1,902 patient visits—initiated conversation to express concerns or specific needs and/or wishes about God. Issues discussed included:

- To die/God to take me
- To know if dead loved one who committed suicide is in hell
- To know where loved one is (heaven, hell, other)
- To know if God has a reason for patient to still be here
- To put situation in hands of the lord/God
- To have God be present
- To know where God is in all this
- To get back to God
- To get spiritual life in order
- To receive answers and miracles

A Summary of Spiritual Care Needs of Patients

Based on the examples provided in this chapter, it can be said that patients have a spiritual need to make choices about what they talk about and to whom they will share what is important to them. Sometimes they want to talk about their health, their relationships, their feelings, and their perceptions of their future. Sometimes they just wish to have a chatty visit and not go deeply into any one thing. All of these types of conversations are spiritually uplifting and significant to some patients. Even the most ordinary conversation can meet spiritual needs for connectedness.

At other times, patients have a need to identify specific services needed and to have these services met. Some of the services desired are based on common needs to talk about spiritual practices and barriers to spiritual development as well as theological matters and issues regarding the patient's relationship to God or other higher power. In these cases, patients expressed their own thoughts and feelings and tried to find some resolution, comfort, or change as a result of their conversation with the chaplain. In situations where a patient does not want to talk to a chaplain, for whatever reason, a respectful response on the chaplain's part can lead to increased feelings of acceptance on the part of the patient. This acceptance can be an outcome in and of itself. It can also lead to a different interaction in the future.

WHAT DO PATIENTS NEED FROM YOU?

In this age of data collection and propensity to engage in surveys, it is possible to come up with a large variety of ways to gather information about what patients want and need from chaplains during the hospitalization process. The important thing is to find a way to gather data and use it to shape the services you provide. For example, one can gain information about the wishes and needs of patients in any number of the following ways:

- Listening (anecdotal)
- Reviewing process notes
- Reviewing service notes of staff and interns
- Keeping lists of requests from patients at morning meetings
- Keeping track from requests in general
- Formalizing patient request forms
- Having periodic focus groups
- Leaving room on satisfaction surveys for wishes and needs not listed
- Surveying literature/research

When information about the needs and wishes of patients are gathered and used properly, patients continue to be the center of treatment and services. After all, health care and pastoral care endeavors are both based on the patients needs. When patients' needs and wishes are determined only by the care provider, treatment becomes less collaborative and therefore less efficient and effective in the long run.

Chapter 3

Health, Healing, Illness, and Recovery

> Even in darkness I will learn to wait for the light, confident that it
> will come to cast its shaft across my path at the point of my great-
> est and most tragic need. Because God is the God of the darkness
> as well as the light, I shall be unafraid of the darkness. I will keep
> my heart open to truth and light. (Thurman, 1953, p. 190)

For many years I have worked in a hospital where a majority of patients have difficulty understanding that they are ill. In fact, they often
feel healthy, even when this is not the case. This lack of insight can
make treatment and recovery even more challenging. This is especially true since mental illness often robs a person of the clarity
needed in processing the reality of that illness. But not all patients are
deprived of such insight into the medical reality of their situation.
Some can be helped to recognize that they have an illness and that
there are treatments available to help them manage it. When this is
the case, the illness does not become the defining factor of who patients are as people.

In addition to mental illness, there are other illnesses that are less evident to persons who have them. Pervasive illnesses such as diabetes,
high blood pressure, excessive stress, and substance addictions are not
always recognized by patients as illnesses. Other diseases such as cancer
and AIDS may lie dormant within a person for quite some time before
one becomes aware of its presence. Once identified, these illnesses are
challenging enough to require time and emotional processing before
true insight and treatment management is possible.

It may be that those who recognize they have an illness, or other
challenge to their health and well-being are the fortunate ones. Many
go to their doctor and seek help. If they need hospitalization, or another type of treatment, they usually take the necessary steps to get it.
After a course of treatment has been planned, implemented, and com-

pleted, many experience recovery and return to a state of health. This return to health is a pleasant state of affairs. Such a belief comes once a successful treatment program has been completed.

THE GIFT OF A 100 PERCENT CURE

I called Sam on a workday. I knew that he was not working as he was between positions. I wanted to tell him that my husband was being scheduled for heart valve replacement surgery and that I needed to take a several month break from committee work. I needed to remove some things from my list of "things to do." It was enough to process at personal and relational levels.

Sam answered the phone promptly. He did not sound good. Something was not right. I told him about taking a break until the first of the year. At that point he said, "You didn't know, I just got through prostate surgery a month ago and am still in recovery. I'm weak and it could take eight or ten weeks to get back to 85 percent of my normal self. It could take a year before I fully recover, if I do fully recover. But the doctor said the surgery went well and that I was 100 percent cured from prostate cancer. They caught it early!"

THEMES OF HEALTH, HEALING, ILLNESS, AND RECOVERY

This chapter focuses on the themes of health, healing, illness, and recovery. These themes shape our basic assumptions and understandings about health care. As such, they inform the way we perceive the needs of hospitalized patients and the services that chaplains and spiritual care providers deliver to patients and to their families.

It is not possible to be engaged in hospital ministry for a period of time without facing questions about health, healing, illness, and recovery. However, it is possible never to have taken sufficient time to develop satisfactory answers to these processes and to provide corresponding helpful services. A caregiver not recently reflecting on these themes and processes is usually due to one of two reasons: certain personality types are "doers" rather than "thinkers"; and in other cases, it is common for caregivers to be so engaged in the "trees" of hospital ministry that they are just too tired to look at the "forest" or the larger picture. In both cases the spiritual caregiver is a "doer," either by nature or out of expediency.

The first part of this chapter is devoted to opening a much-needed discussion about the themes and processes of health, healing, illness, and recovery. The selected questions are divided into areas that are complementary and often clustered together in the health care field. The list of questions considered is not exhaustive, nor is it heavily steeped on the conceptual side. Rather, the purpose of thinking about these questions is to facilitate the thinking and practice of hospital ministry personnel.

The questions considered on the following pages are presented in four groupings:

1. Questions about health and illness
    What is health?
    When does health become illness?
    How have we changed our thinking about health and illness?
2. Questions about wellness and recovery
    How does healing connect with wellness and recovery?
    What is wellness?
    Is there a specific point known as recovery?
3. Questions about healing and hope
    Is healing a physical, mental, or spiritual term?
    What is the role of hope?
    Can one lend hope?
    How does one construct hope?
4. Questions about the role of beliefs
    Do beliefs affect health, illness, and healing?
    Are there beliefs that are more helpful?
    Are there beliefs that are less helpful?

QUESTIONS ABOUT HEALTH AND ILLNESS

Not everyone agrees on what constitutes health, healing, illness, and recovery, or how one determines the point at which these terms are appropriately used to describe a person's condition in life. Furthermore, few health care providers in a hospital setting worry about these questions from a philosophical and conceptual point of view. Those who do ponder these questions are likely to have moved through their profession to become educators, researchers, and writers. Others may also ponder the decisions and treatment that they provide, particularly when faced with difficult treatment issues.

However, when it comes to definitions of health and illness, there is a surprising lack of diversity in the health care field. Chaplains, with their reflective, spiritual care, and counseling stance, often push the envelope of the prevailing medical paradigm concerning health and illness. Patients, families, and other health consumers, also tend to push the medical paradigm in order to meet their needs. Professionals from the disciplines, who have integrated spirituality issues into their health care practice, are also likely to challenge the rest of the hospital community to search for differing and more holistic understandings of health and illness.

What is health?

The words "health" and "healthy" traditionally refer to a somewhat measurable physical condition that is considered normative for a majority of people. A "healthy" person is one who has no illness. This means that all parts and processes of the body are working at optimum capacity, or as close as possible. A person who suffers "ill-health" has one or more physical conditions that either will respond to treatment or keep the person in a state of "ill-health."

According to this thinking, a person suffering from gout, for example, who does not respond to treatment is not in good health. In other cases, parts of one's body such as the appendix, could be taken out and the person can remain in good health since the organ itself is not considered essential to the functioning of the human body. However, the appendix does create a health problem if it is malfunctioning and can cause damage to other parts of the body if it is not removed.

Physical health is a delicately balanced condition that may vary slightly from person to person. In this line of thinking, a healthy body temperature might be 98.6, give or take a degree. Still, a state of healthiness implies that every physical part, at the cellular and organic level, is working reasonably well and in harmony. This is known as the mechanistic model, which had its origins in the latter part of the nineteenth century when medicine and modern biology were growing fields that helped develop much of the basis of practical scientific thinking.

The use of the term "health" to describe physical functioning is so common to all of us that it may seem somewhat strange to lift it up and describe it here. However, this view of health, considered traditional in the western part of the world, has not always been its predominant understanding, nor has its current narrowness remained unchallenged. Still its physical, narrow definition remains functionally predominant in most hospitals.

However, there has been a growing trend toward holistic understandings of "health" which recognizes that physical health alone is not a sign of total "healthiness." Other dimensions of a person can be functioning at less than full working condition. Those who have broadened the term "health" look to normative conditions that constitute emotional, social-relational, and spiritual health in addition to physical well-being. Of course, mental health is now considered by many persons in the field of psychiatry to be primarily a physical function that also affects other functioning systems within an individual. These differing aspects of health take into account how an individual begins life, how a person develops, and the expected and unexpected events that happen throughout one's life. As such, the broader view of health is a relational and contextual view built upon current understandings and complexities of all living beings.

When does health become illness?

During everyone's life there are circumstances that challenge optimum health. When a person experiences a cold or flu, they are said to be "ill." The nose runs, the eyes run, a cough sounds, and the throat may become reddened and irritated. Parts of the body are not in harmony with other parts. Attempts are made to return to a pre "illness" state. From a professional and commonsense point of view, even the common cold is considered an "illness" that renders a person unhealthy, and in a state of functioning not so well.

Traditionally, the words "illness" and "health" have been used mutually exclusively. A person is either healthy or ill. At the same time, most people have come to understand that illness can be at work with or without the person knowing something is not working at optimum level. Also, our modern understanding is that illness can sometimes develop over time or it can occur fairly rapidly. These varying factors make illness difficult to assess and respond to in a timely fashion, even if one knows what remedies are helpful. They also make "health" and "illness" less mutually exclusive terms when combined with other dimensions of emotional, sociorelational, and spiritual functions which have generated much rethinking in many recent health care circles.

How have we changed in our thinking about health and illness?

For thousands of years, health and illness were mainly attributed to the way things were created and how God, or gods, related to human beings. Human health and illness were viewed in terms of our relationship to God, God's will and intentions for humans. As with most things, health and illness were mysteries and everyone knew that God, or a representative of God, was the keeper of the keys to such mysteries. Wondering about the causes and effects of illnesses and health has apparently always been part of the human way of trying to understand ourselves and the world around us.

The Influence of Hebrew and Christian Thinking

On the European and American continent, a Hebrew and Christian worldview has dominated human thought for the past several hundred years, the reference point being sacred Hebrew (Jewish) and Christian scriptures and traditions. This is not to say there was unified thinking about health and illness in these Hebrew and Christian scriptures and traditions, but several threads have been used in hospital ministry, and the training of clergy and chaplains, for the past couple of generations. These threads are:

- God created the world, and everything in it, and it was declared good.
- God made early choices about the possibilities and limits for humans. We did not always follow these choices and limits. Therefore, we have a history of getting into trouble.
- One of the ways trouble shows up in humans is through illness and disease, both natural, and caused by human choices and omissions.
- Remedies for handling trouble, in the form of illness and disease, include: faith, prayer, self-examination, change in spiritual practices, and social and communal changes. Recommended interventions include the use of physical/biological remedies and

tangible resources gleaned from nature and creation (including human ministrations).

- Some illnesses and diseases lead to acute, chronic, and life threatening situations that may include permanent challenges, even death.
- A person with an illness is expected to turn to friends, families, temple and/or church, social resources, and to God, if one wants to move from illness back to a state of health.

The Influence of Western Thinking on Non-Western Views

A modern example of changing worldviews can be found in the following example about health and illness in the Samoan culture. The earliest Samoan worldview is based on an understanding of the role of gods in health and illness. This worldview was greatly influenced by Christian thinking. It is shared here because it is somewhat prototypical as western influence moved into the American continent and throughout large portions of our world.

Example: Changes in the Samoan culture. In the Samoan Islands there co-exists two worldviews pertaining to health and illness. In the "pre-contact medical paradigm," according to MacPherson (1985, pp. 1-15), illness indicated the displeasure of the *aitu* (a generic term for supernatural agents). Interventions to change the ill condition, therefore, included, a review of personal or group behavior. This was necessary because certain behaviors might have offended the *aitu* and been the cause of the illness. Once the *aitu* was appeased through this correction of behavior, the community/individual returned to health. If corrections were not made (or not appropriately made), sickness and eventually death would occur.

Upon contact with European medical models and diseases, it became clear that some illness could not be explained or contained in this worldview. A new pattern of illness was evident and thus new conceptions and interventions were needed. According to MacPherson, it was the missionaries who "introduced the possibility of simultaneous belief in the omnipotence of a deity and a greater role in the management of illness" (MacPherson, 1985, p. 4). After these changes and influences became more pervasive, treatment for illnesses were assigned to appropriate healer or healers after a diagnosis of the situation, assumptions of cause(s), and appreciation of the variety, uniqueness, and potential interaction of various resources was determined.

Within the old and the adapted paradigms remained a core belief that the human condition is normally one of balance and equilibrium. Illness is a disruption of that balance and its restoration is the goal of any intervention. Restoration, therefore, is essential for the individual and for the community.

Current Reconnections of Mind, Body, and Spirit in the Medical World

Attempts to look at the interconnections between mind, body, and spirit abound as we move forward into the twenty-first century. However, the mind, body, and spirit movement of the twenty-first century is built on ancient foundations. Its roots are firmly planted in eastern and western traditions representing diverse, rich experiences. Much of these experiences have been spiritually centered. This is not surprising since ancient wisdom has always looked at the physical world through spiritual eyes.

It has been a brief, recent moment in time that humans have been captivated by a cultural belief that the mind must be separated from the body, and that the body and mind must be considered separate from the spirit. This approach has helped religion and science both grow as mutually exclusive disciplines. This splitting of mind, body, and spirit has been prevalent over the greater part of the last 125 years. This, of course, is the heyday of modern medicine, modern psychology and psychiatry, developing social services, and the growth of modern industry.

But this rift between mind, body, and spirit, is narrowing each day as more and more health care providers and consumers understand the need to bring together all healing resources available if health and healing are to occur. What has brought about these changes is that there are more informed people, specialists if you will, who can attend to the efficacy of differing healing processes. This is a good thing and not to be feared by traditional specialists who focus only on the mind, body, or spirit. For no one person can be an expert to the whole person, but can be skilled in helping a part connect to the whole.

Herbert Benson is one of a number of professionals who promotes this connectedness and thus contributes to changing our views of health and medicine. He is a medical doctor who remains firmly planted in his discipline while reaching out to recapture and renew holistic health care practices. In his book, *Timeless Healing,* he states,

> ... my patients have taught me a great deal about the opportunities that emerge when artificial barriers are broken down, about how physical ailments inspire soul-searching and a revival of meaningful living, and about how the human spirit enlivens and transforms the body. (Benson, 1996, p. 287)

QUESTIONS ABOUT WELLNESS AND RECOVERY

How does healing connect with wellness and recovery?

It is probably not too far-fetched to declare that at one time the Western world assumed that medical advances being made between the nineteenth and twentieth centuries would bring about healing for almost all diseases. That is a goal and hope that still drives most research in the health care field today. It is a worthy goal as long as we understand that goals are guides, not universal truths. The truth is that we humans have limits, and one we all share is birth and death. How far we will be able to push these two elements, however, has yet to be seen.

In the meantime, the practical focus of health care providers, health care chaplains, and pastoral counselors turns to the everyday dilemma of focusing on healing while understanding the limits of restorative health efforts. The truth remains that many persons cannot be restored to the state of youth or function as they were before an illness or health care intervention. Because of this health care reality, new words such as wellness and recovery have been coined to describe how a person can recover and still not function at 100 percent physically, mentally, or spiritually. A person can experience well-being and not meet criteria for a clean bill of mental or physical health.

Margaret Kornfeld, pastoral counselor, author, and president of the American Association of Pastoral Counselors, is an example of a health care provider who understands the dynamic fluidity and interconnectedness of human functioning within given parameters of health, healing, illness, wellness, and recovery. In her recent book, *Cultivating Wholeness,* she writes:

> We are learning that to be healthy does not mean to be symptom-free. We are learning that health is not just the opposite of illness:

Health is the consciousness of one's wholeness—and that means accepting one's limitations as well as one's strengths. We are also learning that we can become aware of our wholeness and still die. We can experience "health" and well-being even though our bodies might have conditions labeled "terminal illness." (Kornfield, 1998, p. 8)

What is wellness?

If wellness is not equivalent to a state of health that demonstrates optimum functioning of mind, body, and spirit, then we must begin to think outside of our mythical superhero boxes. The concept of wellness points us toward hopeful and helpful functioning in the good times as well as the challenging ones. Wellness does not deny the reality of illness nor the desire for optimum health. Instead, it adds a valuing process that pivots around the experience of "self" and "self as meant to be." It is the "self" that can experience wellness of being in the midst of other facets of mind or body that perhaps don't work. It is the "self" that can experience well-being and acceptance in the midst of spiritual ambiguities and questionable life journeys. Wellness, as a health care concept, draws the person, the family, and the community, into a healing process that allows space for all kinds of positive things to happen. In the wellness paradigm there is even room for mystery and miracle.

Is there a specific point known as recovery?

This is a common question for those suffering from substance abuse, chronic mental illness, or a recurring illness such as cancer. The most helpful answer must manage to lend hope, acknowledge progress, affirm current levels of functioning, and leave open our lack of a crystal ball. Recovery, like wellness, is a state of being realistically affirmed as "okay" by the wise and informed. It is founded on faith. It is quite a humbling and profound experience to be able to say, "I believe I have recovered from this health problem and I accept that I can experience well-being."

For most of us it is important to look toward recovery. It is a healthy exercise to be in the process of recovering from any and all obstacles to being our "self" and the "self we were meant to be." Life is process and as such has a natural affinity for health, healing, wellness, and recovery. These processes are life's natural mechanisms for meeting challenges such as illness or disease. The words we use in conceptualizing health care are important pointers to the reality of life that is given to us as a gift from the divine and higher power.

QUESTIONS ABOUT HEALING AND HOPE

It would not be truthful to say that questions of healing and hope are asked by most health care professionals. Certainly the question of healing is raised and certain evidences of healing are paid attention by some in health care. But more and more professionals are now addressing the role of hope and the questions concerning the healing of the whole human being. These questions should be everyone's concern and not just the interest of health care chaplains and pastoral counselors.

Is healing a physical, mental, or spiritual term?

Healing refers to all processes that move toward one optimum function (health) and toward being the person one is created, called, and meant to be (wellness and well-being). Healing refers to the processes at work internally within persons, and externally within relationships. These processes of healing are brought about naturally, by divine intervention and plans, and through specific planned and unplanned human interventions. Healing involves living processes within living beings and can be said to have taken place once life changes have been observed. These observations may be both subjective and objective though it is not safe to assume, however, that if healing occurs in the physical sense it is also completed in the mental or spiritual sense, or vice versa. It does follow that real healing yearns for completeness in all areas of life.

What is the role of hope?

Hope was a common word in the experiences of ancient Hebrew people and it is documented throughout their scriptures. It was also found in the Christian letters of the Apostle Paul. Hope is observed by Paul to be an affective state that leads to motivated action through life giving processes. Like healing, hope moves us forward into being.

In Paul's letter to the Romans, he considers the issue of "sufferings of this present time" (8:18) and looks forward to the salvation of all humankind from the "groaning travail" (8:22) that the children of God now face. The way through suffering and travail, for Paul, was through the process he refers to as "hope." In Chapter 8:24-25, Paul defines and describes what he means by "hope":

> For in this hope we were saved. Now hope that is seen is not hope. For who hopes for what he sees? But if we hope for what we do not see, we wait for it with patience. (RSV)

Christian hope, according to Paul, leads us through physical, emotional, and spiritual problems, and through our grief (groaning travails) concerning these problems. In this sense, hope is an energizing and motivationally affective state that leads to movement, process, and change. Hope, as an energizer and motivator, is generated by the divine spirit that dwells within the human spirit. Hence, we don't see it. We don't really have a complete definition of it. We can only allude to hope by observing its process, much as we observe the process of faith.

The end product of hope, for Paul, was salvation. So, what can be seen from the activity of hope is a movement away from separation and fragmentation toward life-giving wholeness. From a health care perspective, we can see the parallel ways in which hope points us toward health, healing, and wellness. Just as spiritual hope in the reality of salvation leads us toward that end, so too does spiritual hope in the reality of health, healing, and recovery lead us toward present day experiences of salvation (self as we are meant to be).

Can one lend hope?

Another fruit of hope, in addition to salvation from suffering and travail, is patience. This is crucial to healing and health care processes and it can take time and involve time-consuming interventions. One of the ways Christians can fulfill the commandment of Jesus to "Heal the sick" (Matthew 10:8), is by looking for kernels of hope in all situations and persons, and by lending one's own hope to those who do not currently have access to their own. This lending of hope is a task undertaken by all health care professionals, but it is one of the prime tasks of chaplains and spiritual care providers.

One can lend hope to another person in many ways. To begin with, it is an act of hope for a caregiver to explore and practice ways of fostering hope in others. It takes both time and patience to lend and be filled with the spirit of hope in the presence of one who may be feeling hopeless. In hospital ministry, we lend hope in many of the following ways:

- Affirmation of treatment options and interventions
- Helping to sort out choices based on personal values
- Efforts toward promoting qualities of self-esteem, dignity, patient rights
- Helping the person to wonder about things with a spirit of humility
- Referring to mysteries and opening up the possibility that God or a divine power may be working on the situation
- Offering to pray with someone or on someone's behalf
- Explicitly talking about hope and what is hoped for
- Sharing knowledge about the strengths of the hospital/staff
- In recurring situations reminding the person of their past healing experiences
- Helping a person discover their strengths and identify coping options and resources
- Letting the person know that you respect their feelings of hopelessness and at the same time tell them that you prefer to remain hopeful

How does one construct hope?

In *Hope in Pastoral Care and Counseling,* Andrew Lester writes:

> When speaking of hope, I am addressing the configuration of cognitive and affective responses to life that believes the future is filled with possibilities and offers a blessing. Used theologically, the word hope describes a person's trusting anticipation of the future based on an understanding of a God who is trustworthy and who calls us into an open-ended future. (Lester, 1995, p. 62)

Lester goes on to state that he believes hope develops as we project "ourselves into the future dimension by developing future stories . . ." (Lester, 1995, p. 63). The construction of hope, as Lester sees it, is best built through the narratives we develop which tell the stories of who we are and where we feel we are going.

However, it can also be said that hope is not built only on narrative processes such as words, conversation, artistic stories, or actions taken.

Our future stories are probably built into us (hard wired) and are being built as we go along. To a certain degree we develop our own forms of hope that, once created, have infinite capabilities for constructing hope on multiple levels, simultaneously.

One of the dilemmas about the construction of hope, our future, is that we are all products of our genetics development. In light of this, we often construct hope through the righting and balancing, and sometimes the letting go, of excess and unhelpful experiences, thoughts and feelings. To make changes in our experiences of hope we may want to direct ourselves and others through the use of open ended questions such as:

- What would have to be in place for you to be hopeful?
- What would you like to have happen?
- Consider—What/who do you trust?
- If you were building a path to the future what would be some of your first steps?
- What did your family teach you about hope?

Hope is part of our spirit-filled capacity to move into the future. It comes to us at birth, and grows and develops as we journey through life. In that sense it is constructed and becomes part of the construction we call "our lives." But it is never finished nor fully known to any one person. There is always more hope to be had in any life or situation. It is a crucial task of every spiritual care provider, clergy, and chaplain to be in the business of building hope.

THE ROLE OF BELIEFS

Do beliefs affect health, illness, and healing?

Harold Koenig, in his book *Is Religion Good for Your Health?* (1997), concludes, "In general, devout religiousness and frequent involvement in both private and public religious activities are associated with better mental health" (p. 101). Further research also shows that "the effects of religious beliefs and activities on physical health are similar to those on mental health. In general, persons who are religiously involved are healthier than those who are not" (pp. 102-103). As to the neurotic and pathological uses of religion, Koenig states that these "are not widespread nor characteristic of the vast majority of Americans who are religious" (p. 104).

Are there beliefs that are more helpful?

There has been renewed interest in the effects of religion and beliefs on health and healing. Professionals such as Larry Dossey speak of the positive effects that prayer can have on the healing process. In his workshops, he frequently tells of his current practice of praying with patients before surgery, and how current research concerning the power of prayer has changed his way of doing business as a physician. Further information and research about the power of prayer can be found in Dossey's books, including *Healing Words: The Power of Prayer and the Practice of Medicine* (1993).

There is ample research available to demonstrate the power of prayer in promoting health and healing. However, common sense causes many who are hospitalized to seek the practice of prayer as a personal spiritual care practice, and as a healing tool employed by chaplains and others in an intercessory manner. Other beliefs that involve imaging and devotional reading are believed to be efficacious by many persons who are hospitalized. Some believe that Holy Communion is important to healing processes. Of course, there are ample numbers of Americans who have been influenced by Norman Vincent Peale's *The Power of Positive Thinking,* and will be heard saying to self and others, "Keep a good thought, things will get better." Prayer was considered by Dr. Peale to be one of the most helpful of good thoughts as he first published this book in the 1950s.

According to Herbert Benson, another physician and researcher in the field of mind, body, and spirit and the effects of religion on the health of the body and person,

> . . . I have been continually amazed to see that beliefs do generate these kinds of quantifiable results. Nevertheless, I don't want to denigrate the subjective—what people think and feel. . . . Beliefs manifest themselves differently in the body, and while some beliefs bring about results the professions can measure . . . others produce symptoms that are real in their effect on patients but perhaps cannot be tracked down . . . (Benson, 1996, p. 29)

Are there beliefs that are less helpful?

According to Harold Koenig (1997),

> Primary care physicians and other medical professionals, while less forceful in their negative opinions of religion's influences than their psychiatric colleagues, nevertheless largely see religion as irrelevant to health and the delivery of good health care. (p. 30)

Health care providers in the field of psychiatry have had more exposure to the difficulties patients have in processing religious material and their personal beliefs while under psychotic influences and some mental illnesses. It is common for some professionals in psychiatric hospitals to spend more time looking at the pathological beliefs a patient may have during an acute episode of a mental disorder. This has often led to neglect or inattention to religious and spiritual beliefs in many cases.

Again, common sense and experience in the chaplaincy field has shown that some beliefs are less helpful to individuals seeking healing. One of the most frequent beliefs presenting an obstacle to healing is known as fatalism. Fatalism combined with its consequent feelings of hopelessness and helplessness often leads to a narrowing of options and choices. The more a fatalistic belief is globalized, the greater chance that belief has at becoming an obstacle to health and healing.

THE DEVELOPMENT OF CORE IMAGES OF HEALTH AND ILLNESS

Core images are those experience-reflections that remain long after individual experiences of health and illness have passed. By listening for continuing themes, metaphors, and statements about health and illness, we are able to hear patients better. Furthermore, by engaging in this collaborative imaging process we are better able to assist patients in their recovery processes.

Core images about health and illness can be very powerful predictors of the healing outcomes of health care interventions. This is so because everyone has their own unique viewpoint and puts together personal imagery around their own health, illness, and recovery.

These core health images may come out in a number of ways. They may be stated directly in story, metaphor, or in parable. They may be found in changes of expression, body posture, and movement. They may be found in the types of music listened to, material read, and in relationships. These health images are also found in the way treatment is discussed, in philosophical statements made about life in general, and in reflections of the specifics of one's life. Core images of health and healing are also found in the content of prayers and in the choice and use of devotional and sacred writings.

For an image to be a core image it must have an internal correspondence to the meaning that a person ascribes his or her life, health, healing, and illness. For inner correspondence to happen, an inner connectedness must occur involving three or more areas within the person: physical, mental, emotional, social, and/or spiritual. In most cases a core image involves all five areas, or the whole person.

Finding Core Images of Health, Healing, and Illness

The best way to discover the nature and depth of a patient's image of health, healing, and illness is to reflect on what the person says about these things. We can do so by directing the conversation, and we can reflect on what we have seen and heard as a conversation progresses unimpeded. In the following section, six patients talk about their diseases. Their thoughts and feelings present a poignant picture of how they view their illness and hospitalization process. As one reads through these stories, one is able to access the depths of personal experience which are likely to be a part of the practice of hospital ministry.

Experiences and Reflections of Patients Who Have Severe Illnesses

Severe Back Pain

I can't do the things I used to do, so I have to ask for help. I'm not used to that. But that's how it works when you are disabled. I don't get out much anymore, not like I used to be able to do. I have to rely on my parents and that puts a strain on them and on me. I miss my friends but they have their own lives. I just hate not being able to work and get around without all this pain. It's just not acceptable.

Advanced Cancer

I had to come in because I was falling quite a lot. There was no one nearby who could stay with me. I've lived in my home most of my life, and now I don't know what is going to happen to it or me. I just can't seem to keep from crying. I'm sorry. Yesterday the doctor said I have cancer throughout my body. I'm scared. The chaplain came by but I just can't seem to get comfortable and I couldn't take communion. Maybe later. I don't want to die. Like I said, the doctors still don't know what's going to happen to me.

Cardiac Problem

When I came in I was in so much pain. I knew I wasn't going to make it. I remember just laying there and praying to God to help me through it. I prayed that it be God's will that I make it. I wouldn't let myself think of dying. I have lots I want to do in life. My family and the doctors are encouraged by my overall improvement this past week. I just knew my prayers were stronger than that heart attack. It just goes to show you what prayer can do.

Experiences and Reflections of Patients Who Have Mental Illness

Being Hospitalized for the First Time

I made a mistake. Everything seems to be going wrong. I don't belong here, I'm really scared. You don't know what it's like to be here. People are really sick. There's yelling and screaming. The other patient in my room keeps me up all night. I can't believe my family did this to me. I can't take a shower alone. I can't go outside. They expect me to cope but my inner resources are depleted. Coercion is not going to change that. They've taken away my freedom. That's what I've lost, my freedom!

Being Diagnosed with Bipolar Disorder

They say I have a mental illness. I'm not sure. They say I have to take this medication but it makes me drowsy and I don't want to do things. I miss having the energy I used to have. They say I don't have much depression but I tend to be manic. I like being energetic. I got so much done when I was energetic. I made money and had all kinds of interesting projects. I went everywhere. In fact, the people I used to work for say they want me back as soon as I'm out of the hospital. My family has more problems with this than I do. I don't care what they say; they have the keys and I'm suffering in here.

Suffering from Major Depression

It just comes over me and I can't seem to do anything. I want to die. I just pray that God will take me. Why does he make me suffer? I sleep all day. I don't have the energy to get up. They brought me back here because I wasn't taking my meds and I missed a doctor's appointment. I don't care. I can't even think of anything but dying. The only reason I try not to kill myself is because of my kids. That's just not a good thing to do to them.

IMAGES OF HEALTH AND ILLNESS

When an individual discovers that she or he has an illness, there is a natural reaction of grief. The person goes through stages of shock, denial, emotions, and depression, and struggles to reorganize temporarily around the tasks related to recovery. This process is true whether it's another bout of the common cold or something more challenging such as a biopsy or the need for major surgery. Depending on the nature of the illness, the grieving may be brief or it may continue for a lengthy period of time, as is often the case with major and/or chronic illnesses.

Grief and recovery involve numerous aspects such as images of the nature of the illness/problem, the resources available, the prognosis and type of recovery expected, thoughts and feelings about the cause of the illness, and the role one presumes to have played or not played in the development of the illness. Another factor in the course of grieving and the individual's response to an illness, is the image that emerges and is attached to the illness. Often this imagery gives the illness added meaning.

About Images

All people use images consciously and unconsciously to express clusters or constellations of thoughts, feelings and experiences. Once clustered, these images are ascribed a specific meaning. As a rule images include:

- Vivid portrayals and descriptions in language form
- Mental pictures
- Representations—loose, repetitious, and ordinary
- Symbolic representations

People differ as to their use and preference of differing types of images. Those who are visually oriented, for example, may have more mental pictures come to them. Those who are more auditory and verbal may use specific phrases and other language act as imagery. Others may find they readily respond to symbolic representations or other associations that may not reach a specific symbolic form.

Images of health and illness vary in intensity, pervasiveness, and in the effect they have on an individuals' health and healing. Each image can be reviewed according to type, specific image, content, and ascribed meaning. The intensity range can be from mild to moderate, strong, or extreme. The pervasiveness of the image can be limited, partially expanded, generalized, or global. The effect an image has on health and healing can range from constructive to challenging, to potentially harmful, or destructive. These imagery classifications are noted in Table 3.1.

TYPES OF IMAGES ENCOUNTERED
IN TREATMENT OF PATIENTS

Five types of commonly held imagery can be labeled in ways that describe their function in the lives of most patients. In this sense they

TABLE 3.1. Classification of Health and Illness Images

Image	Intensity	Pervasiveness	Effect
Type	Mild	Limited	Constructive
Specific image	Moderate	Partially Expanded	Challenging
Content	Strong	Generalized	Potentially Harmful
Ascribed Meaning	Extreme	Global	Destructive

Note: Chart reads from top to bottom in each column, not from left to right.

are generalized. Their description is followed by a vignette/example. The five commonly held images are:

1. Scene recall imagery
2. Personified attribute imagery
3. Meaning pocket imagery
4. Nebulous imagery and loose representations
5. Multiple imagery constellations

Scene Recall Imagery

Included under this grouping are memory flashbacks and/or intrusions and pictorial associations that may come from sources other than personal memory. These sources might be written material, cultural images, and images from the media. Scene recall images may also include dissociative material that comes from the unconscious and that the individual does not have direct conscious access or control over. Imagery in this category adhere to the classification of health and illness images found in Table 3.1. Hence, their power and effect varies accordingly.

Example

Tina lost her mother six months ago and had been experiencing vivid recall of her mother in memories and what she called "visions." She would sometimes see her mother coming toward her and she would have a waking conversation with this vision. With help, she learned that some of what she was experiencing was typical for persons who had lost loved ones who they were intensely close to. She also knew that some aspects of her "dead mother" visions might be tied up in her mood disorder. In addition, she had very vivid images of special times with her mother. In general, these memory-laden images were of comfort to her, even though they were painful in her grieving process.

Tina's imagery consisted of vivid descriptions and mental pictures with perhaps some unknown mystery involved. She always said, "I am a very spiritual person." There also may have been some distortion of reality due to the combination of her grieving and mood disorder. The intensity of these images ranged from strong to extreme at the time of her pastoral counseling intervention. On her good days, Tina could see that her illness affected her grieving and her health, and she could see how the illness worsened during her most difficult times. At other times she was able to see the grieving combined with her illness as pervasive but not without hope of recovery. The effect of the visions and memories was mostly to promote healing. However, during her most difficult periods of illness, her desire to die became a potentially destructive component that made her grieving and recovery more difficult.

Another Example

Brian greatly dreaded his upcoming heart surgery. He couldn't get over notions that the surgery might turn out okay, but that he might become very disabled as a result, and be confined to the living room couch, unable to live the quality of life he felt he deserved. Whenever friends and loved one's brought up the impending surgery, Brian minimized his responses, which only made his relationships more stressed. Finally, just before the surgery, Brian spoke with a chaplain who asked him about how he pictured his recovery progressing. This gave Brian the opportunity to talk about an image that kept coming to him about what had happened to his grandfather. Brian confessed that he could not think of the surgery without picturing his grandfather taking to the couch, and for all practical purposes, declaring himself an old man with a bad heart and staying there until he died. Once the image was shared, Brian sheepishly stated that he felt some relief, by just getting it off his chest.

Brian had what can be described as scene recall image. This image connected his grandfather's heart surgery to his own impending surgery. The intensity of this recalled image was strong, although not extreme. Its pervasiveness was partially expanded and stood a chance of becoming generalized. The image did not keep Brian from having surgery, but the outcome and recovery were effective. Had the image remained so intense it might have proved potentially harmful in its silent and hidden form.

Personified Attribute Imagery

At times a patient will have an image that does not come from personal memory or from a specific scene. These images about health and illness are usually instances where some abstract attribute is attached to health or illness, and the combined association becomes personified as though it had a life similar to a human being. The personified images may be mental pictures, symbolic representations, and/or vivid descriptions.

Example

After being in the psychiatric unit for three days and having a battery of tests and interviews from team members, Billy was confronted with the fact that the team believed he had bipolar disorder. Billy was in his twenties and became quite enraged at the thought of having a mental illness. He began immediately to use words such as "fight," "win," and "defeat." He began to talk about the team as "them." When group leaders wondered about all this increased anger and battle imagery, their observations were confirmed by Billy who declared, "You're damn right. This is a battle and they are the enemy. No way am I going to let this destroy me. I'm going to fight them and I'm going to win."

This image of battle and enemy hindered Billy's ability to constructively meet the challenge of mental illness. Some of the challenge was partly the nature of this type of illness and that of denial and anger stages of grief. However, it turned out that Billy saw himself as young and strong, somewhat of a knight in shining armor who had the whole world as his oyster. The attributes of strength and being right and just overrode attributes of weakness and victim, and other less positive attributes that he ascribed to "sick" people.

Meaning Pocket Imagery

In times of difficulty people naturally look for meaning and purpose. On most occasions the search for meaning is one that springs from the depths of hope that sparks all living things, and seems to be part of our creator's original design. Sometimes, however, the meaning and purpose experienced in life can be more negative than positive, more malevolent than benign or benevolent. When meaning and purposes of health, healing, and recovery are imaged in the positive, the person experiences hope. When this is not true the lack of positive meaning and purpose can lead to despairing spiritual images.

Example

As I began writing the first draft of this chapter my husband, John, was preparing for heart surgery. He needed an aortic valve replacement. We are both chaplains. He works in a general hospital near Boston and I work in a psychiatric hospital in New Hampshire. We were both in shock and just a bit scared. At 5:00 a.m. on the day of the surgery we arrived at Catholic Medical Center and my husband was prepared for surgery. As luck would have it, we waited until 10:15 for John to be taken to surgery. He went his way and I went to sit and wait.

At preadmission the day before I had asked that Sister Andrea be contacted from the pastoral care department. We had not been able to touch base that day. I was tired and somewhat insulated for the first two hours. The cardiac waiting room was filled to capacity and smelled overwhelmingly of perfume. I chose to wait in some chairs outside. The sounds in the hall were loud as the elevators were going up and down all morning. Within the first hour I began to become overwhelmed and wished I had a chaplain. The tears started to build and my thoughts turned immediately to the chapel. I went there. There in the back of the chapel I began to cry. The fact that this was an obviously Catholic chapel made no difference. It was filled with meaning and hope for me in a troubled time.

As the tears subsided I reached for the Bible in the pew. Scanning the scriptural themes I found Isaiah 35:4-7.

> Thus says the Lord:
> Say to those whose hearts are frightened:
> Be strong, fear not!
> Here is your God,
> he comes with vindication;
> with divine recompense
> he comes to save you.
> Then will the eyes of the blind be opened,
> the ears of the deaf be cleared;
> then will the lame leap like a stag,
> then the tongue of the mute will sing.
> Streams will burst forth in the desert,
> and rivers in the steppe.
> The burning sands will become pools,
> and the thirsty ground, springs of water.

To me, this scripture corresponded immediately to my husband's heart condition, and to my own feelings of fright and hurt. I focused on "frightened heart," and "to save," and found some comfort in the image of God's healing. If the eyes of the blind would be opened, and the ears of the deaf cleared, then I needed to trust that John's heart would be made well again. The chapel, the presence of a chaplain somewhere in the facility, the words of scripture, were all part of the meaning pocket that I imagined held the healing component to John's situation. A room with symbols, a woman with call, training, and four sentences became a meaning pocket that held the image of healing and well-being. Each part was a carrier of interpretation for what was happening spiritually in the midst of this operation. As I left the chapel, I wrote a prayer on a slip of paper and placed it in the container marked "prayer intentions." I felt better.

Back in the waiting area, I continued to be hypervigilant, and was irritated by any and all noises. I tried to read my book. A chaplain friend of John's, Ann, stopped by. I was so pleased to see her. She sat with me for some time. Then she left and I got some lunch.

Ann came back and sat with me during the last of the four hours of waiting. She offered to pray. I wanted her to, but did not want to ask. She was there when the doctor came and said the surgery had gone well and that John would be going into recovery. About fifteen minutes later Sister Andrea came and stayed with me. She graciously checked on what was happening in intensive care. I felt so cared for by these two chaplains.

Nebulous Imagery and Loose Representations

Often, health-related imagery consists of clusters, fragments of phrases, associated memories, less constellated feelings, and effects of any number of these. In cases where this kind of imagery is prevalent, the individual may have a sense of something that he or she can't seem to put together and that relates to the illness and/or the recovery. In some cases the individual takes a certain stance which becomes a living image based on such feelings and thoughts.

Example

His birthday was coming up in a few days. He would be thirty-three. His mind wandered as he talked about symbols in *The National Enquirer,* and trying to see through paper circles. His thoughts moved to things made in the U.S.A., to the numbers 666 and their meaning, and to his desire and search for power. As others were talking about their week and how they were currently doing, he turned back to his age and his birthday, saying, "It's like an air pocket over my head. Everything just floats by."

Multiple Imagery Constellations

Often, health and illness images can consist of combinations of numerous forms of individual imagery. This is so because health and illness images have developed over a long period of time and are stored in numerous ways within the individual. Such imagery may appear to be contradictory at first glance. More than likely, it represents an ambivalency that a person might typically feel.

EFFECTS OF IMAGES ON HEALTH AND ILLNESS

The study of imagery is very useful in devising interventions that are most likely to be effective in promoting health and healing. Once one is able to identify how imagery is being used by a patient and/or his or her family, one has a better chance of assessing its impact on the healing process. Once an assessment is made, a care plan can be devised in collaboration with the patient. In cases where an image is helpful, every effort must be made to employ that image to the benefit of the person. At the other extreme, images that are discovered to have a destructive effect on healthy living can be examined further and processed in such a way that make them lose their potency in the person's life.

Table 3.2 describes a typical continuum of health and illness imagery and their effects on people in general. Imagery are not categorized according to content so much as to their effects.

Categories include:

- Constructive imagery
- Challenging imagery
- Potentially harmful imagery
- Destructive imagery

TABLE 3.2. Images and Their Effects on Health and Illness

Constructive	Challenging	Potentially Harmful	Destructive
A crisis	A destructive force	Enemy	Destroyer
An event	A problem	Fates and chance in capricious, negative action against person	Vengeful God or power
A challenge	A test or trial	Losing a test/trial from God, Satan	The battle lost
Choices	Result of sin, not living right, doing bad	Unworthiness of self	Self as intrinsically bad
Signs of change	Overwhelming cloud	Pervasive and intrusive changes	Whole world collapsing
Natural part of being human	Reminder of frailty of the flesh and order of universe	Bad things happening to good people	Creative design error

Constructive Images of Health and Illness

Constructive images of health and illness are not just naïve or Pollyannaish worldviews. Rather, they are based on realistic understandings of the health care event or crisis. In a sense, these images provide models for individuals to draw strength during a health care crisis/event. Constructive images help create room for choices and for processing change.

Example

Sheila is seventy-nine years old and is losing her eyesight and has a bad heart. She has just had a third heart surgery. She lives alone and is scared. Her daughter has just left the hospital room after telling her that she sees no way that Sheila can go back home. Sheila is alone, afraid, and starts to cry. Later that evening she has a very strong memory of something like this happening to her own mother, Doris. She remembers visiting her mother after her second hip replacement surgery. She remembers her mother fighting off the tears as she declared, "My doctor says I can no longer manage such a large house by myself and that I need to make some decisions. At first I was angry and cried all through the night last night. Then I realized that I could do this. I hate change. I'll miss my home, but I have to do this now while I can do it of my own volition."

Sheila had an image of her mother who was also hospitalized. In this case the image can be called constructive in that a specific scene is recalled by Shelia and used to help her in her current situation. A specific image such as this one is usually self-evident to the patient and often requires little more than a listening affirmation of the crisis, challenge, choices, and change involved.

In some situations, just a simple note of wonder after listening to a patient relate such an image can help the person understand and integrate it into his or her own life. In other circumstances, a person may need help seeing the choices available to him or her. Help may also be needed to process normal feelings of grief that come with changes and/or crisis. The imagery, in this example, is sort of a connector through time and is often seen as a gift or blessing.

Challenging Images of Health and Illness

Imagery becomes challenging when it provokes a prevailing, lingering negative response that presents additional symptoms of increased anxiety and maybe slight depression. As noted in Table 3.2, a challenging image is one that often feels overwhelming or is perceived as coming from an external force. Often, such imagery can have a kind of snowball effect on internal processing, decision-making, and compliance with treatment.

Example

Dan is fifty-four and has been hospitalized numerous times for clinical depression resulting from noncompliance with his prescribed medication, his drinking, and his involvement with nonprescription drugs. He belongs to a conservative church. Every time he faces his noncompliance, drug, and alcohol addictions, he places his head in his hands and begins quoting scripture. He seems to think he is on trial, and is of "weak flesh." However, no matter how much the church and the Word of God come to mind, Dan just can't seem to make changes in his life. Even when he is forced to take medication and does not have access to alcohol or drugs, he cannot put aside the belief that he is being tested by God and that he has sinned. What's more, this sense of being tested and of sinning doesn't seem to motivate him to change. But the images of the church and the words of scripture keep coming to him anyway.

Challenging imagery is not necessarily bad for individuals, however, interventions are usually needed to help assess, understand and process these images. These images can be comforting because they usually help the person make sense of what is happening to them. In this sense, challenging images are similar to constructive images. But, challenging images often require more work to resolve. This is probably so because challenging imagery is presented in problematic terms. Therefore, helping the individual define the problem created by the health care crisis/event is often a good first step. This can be followed by a processing of beliefs and values in the example just discussed. From here on, one can introduce the idea that change is a skill-based process and that learning can take time, effort, and resources.

Potentially Destructive Images of Health and Illness

Potentially harmful images are usually identified by their traumatic feel and descriptions. These images seem to be more globalized, more intense, and sometimes feel potentially more intrusive. Possibly harmful imagery is often recognized by the potentially negative outcomes or consequences implied in the imagery.

Example

Susan was diagnosed with breast cancer and had to have a radical mastectomy. Two years later she was bleeding profusely and ended up, after much testing, having a hysterectomy. She was thirty-two when she had the hysterectomy. She wanted to have more children and now this option was no longer available. Soon after the hysterectomy she started having vivid dreams wherein the same thing always happened. She dreamed she was in the hospital and that she was covered with ugly sores and that there were babies outside the door that she was told she could not touch because she was unclean. Over her bed was this huge crucifix that would suddenly fall on her and crush her. The dream persisted for months. She was still having the dream when she came to the hospital for the removal of a benign cyst on her remaining breast. She had not wanted the surgery and was terrified. She asked to see a priest before submitting to the biopsy.

Imagery often comes in the form of dreams as well as daytime experiences. Again, the destructive, persistent, and painful nature of Susan's dream-imagery makes it potentially harmful. In situations such as this, a chaplain can do best by listening to Susan and helping her express her pain. If the priest should find that Susan is feeling guilty and expresses a desire for confession, sometimes a sacrament is helpful. It would make good clinical sense to refer Susan to a pastoral counselor. Dream imagery does not necessarily need a counselor who is skilled in analytical dream work, but it does require someone who can pay attention to unconscious as well as conscious material. In cases such as Susan's, counseling would be best suggested after the biopsy when discharge is discussed. Therefore, the priest who visits prior to the biopsy would want to suggest a second session down the road.

Destructive Images of Health and Illness

Destructive imagery is identified as that which is likely to lead an individual to take action(s) that a reasonable person would not deem helpful in their recovery. Destructive imagery almost always interferes with health and healing efforts if it is not identified, interpreted, and processed. Often, this means confronting the imagery while still supporting the individual. Destructive imagery is not to be confused with psychotic imagery, since imagery can be destructive and not originate from psychotic origins within the brain. Sometimes it is difficult to separate destructive imagery from imagery gathered from sacred scriptures.

Example

In the mid-1800s, a group of followers from a religious tradition went into the mountains. Everyone in the group expected the second coming of Jesus to happen that day. The day passed and Jesus did not come. Some of the group went home and decided to recalculate the second coming (a constructive approach). Others became intensely sad and some had to be hospitalized for depression (a challenging and potentially harmful approach). One man was admitted to a hospital because he began to think he was Christ and went around telling everyone this was so (a potentially harmful and destructive image).

Health crises come in all shapes and forms. Most of these crises occur outside the hospital and are well in process, with all associated imagery, long before a person enters the hospital. For this reason, one of the most challenging aspects of chaplaincy work is getting as much history surrounding an event as possible in an often severely limited amount of time. Imagery helps chaplains do this more effectively. Destructive images are not always as dramatic as the preceding example but, to be removed as obstacles to health and healing, they always need to have skilled interventions. The rule of thumb with destructive imagery is to establish a positive helping relationship as quickly as possible. Interventions made must be practical, small, and sequential. Referrals are almost always necessary.

In Summary

According to Chris Schlauch, "Every event has a surplus of meaning, in part because it is experienced across so many dimensions—in terms of images, voices, memories, feelings, sensations, and words—in mind and body" (Schlauch, 1995, p. 141). Because this is so, it is crucial for persons engaged in hospital ministry to understand the event known as "hospitalization," and the meanings generated and associated with this event. Often, all of these associated event-meanings are found in the images patients use to describe their thoughts, feelings, beliefs, and experiences. Working with such images, one can assess how a patient is understanding his or her illness and health issues, and help that person take necessary steps to move toward healing and recovery with a greater sense of well-being.

Chapter 4

Establishing a Vision and a Mission for Hospital Ministry

> If vision is a field, think about what we could do differently to use its formative influence. We would start by recognizing that in creating a vision, we are creating a power, not a place, an influence, not a destination. (Wheatley, 1999, p. 55)

In the early 1990s, New Hampshire Hospital in Concord began to explore and engage in self-improvement. A consultant was hired, and 100 upper and middle managers were trained in total quality improvement concepts. The hospital took to the process like a duck to water, and soon, continuous quality improvement became a standard hospital process. A quality council was formed and improvement teams flourished. The process was also integrated hospital-wide at departmental levels. The department of pastoral services was all of a sudden engaged in improvement processes within the department, and participated in multidisciplinary improvement teams.

This was a long way from my early days of working at the Youth Development Center where there were no department, no computers, and no teams. It was also a long way from the early days of hospital ministry which tended to predominately center around the values, vision, ministry style, and focus of each individual chaplain. Still, most pastoral and chaplaincy services have remained essentially unchanged over the years; however, the way in which one gathers information and determines services has changed, and the need to be able to demonstrate outcomes derived from these services has greatly increased.

ASSUMPTIONS AND VALUES

When individuals decide to engage in hospital ministry, they bring to that decision some basic assumptions concerning the nature of such a ministry including: the functions they will perform and for whom; how the functions will be performed; and why they intend to engage in hospital ministry. The question of "why hospital ministry exists at all" may also be contemplated by hospitals and individuals whenever a new employee is being considered.

Interviews for chaplains' positions may be conducted by hospital personnel, directors of pastoral care departments, or by religious group representatives. From the beginning of the initial interview, it is judged whether the assumptions and values of the chaplain-candidate meet those of the health care organization. When there are other pastoral and spiritual care personnel on staff, these persons also bring their assumptions and values that are set in motion during the interview process. The person chosen for the job will be one who the organization, or its representatives, feel is best suited to match the values of the hospital and perhaps its surrounding religious and cultural community.

Unconscious, implicit, distorted, and/or idealized assumptions and values can make the task of choosing a person for a chaplaincy position quite difficult. To add to this challenge, many people don't realize that there are multiple assumptions about hospital ministry, to say nothing of hospital and health care services. Furthermore, seldom does an organization have a single fundamental view governing its actions, nor is it likely that persons in pastoral care and chaplaincy departments will have essentially similar values and views that govern their actions. For these reasons, individuals, departments, and hospitals are encouraged to establish explicit vision and mission statements so that communication and services will both be enhanced.

One Pastoral Care Department's Experience

An acute care psychiatric hospital had a pastoral services department for many years. At one time the department consisted of three full-time and four part-time chaplains. In addition, there was a clinical pastoral education program and a part-time secretary. As the move toward deinstitutionalization of persons with mental illness continued at full force in the late 1970s and early 1980s, the number of patients dwindled, and part-time pastoral staff were let go. However, well into the mid-1990s, three full-time chaplains remained.

In the early 1990s, the hospital began to shift away from clinical pastoral education due to lack of availability of room and board for students. Instead, the department focused on pastoral counseling training. All members of the department were in agreement with this shift, or so it seemed.

Each year, members of the department would gather to look at the previous year's achievements and set new goals for the upcoming year. Many times, two of the three chaplains would focus on clinical care groups, student training, connections with other chaplains, and with general improvement procedures required by the hospital while the third chaplain focused on social efforts and friendly visibility with staff. There was usually room for a bit of everything in the planning process, but goal-setting, and the determination of yearly accomplishments and improvement, made the process increasingly difficult. In many ways, the department was highly functional, and in other ways, it was less than optimally effective due to fundamentally differing assumptions of what services and functions were of most value. The situation was amicable but never really optimized, for each individual valued only his or her point of view.

Value Definition

Values are a subjective way in which we assign worth, importance, and desirability to a concept, feeling, action, or a way of being. We may value many things such as money, clothes, or various body shapes. We often value certain feelings more than others. Most of us value love, faith, and happiness more than we value pain, misery, and feelings of hopelessness. As a culture, we tend to value certain attributes and actions such as hard work, timeliness, and ambition. We do not value laziness, dropping out of high school, or being without a job during what are thought to be working years. We value certain states of being such as sereneness and calmness, meditation, worship, and prayerful living. We do not value couch potato living, aimlessness, and fragmented lifestyles. These are all personal values that are usually learned in contexts of family, school, church, or other organizations. What is valued is often pursued, and what is less valued is often overlooked, avoided, or devalued.

When persons meet in relational gatherings, whether informal or in carefully organized systems, they bring in their personal subjective values with them and put forward those they consider worthy, important, or desirable. As each person brings his or her values to the table, shared values are embraced while those that are not are either pursued individually or placed in positions of less importance. At an organizational level, shared values are often lifted up to become "a principle, standard, or quality considered worthwhile or desirable" (*The American Heritage Dictionary of the English Language* 1973, p. 1414).

Words of Wisdom About Values

As one engages in hospital ministry for an extended period of time, one collects a certain amount of practical wisdom about values as they exist in health care organizations. The sharing of this wisdom can be quite valuable to those who are new to the field. It can also be valuable to those who may find themselves puzzled or continually stepping into "value potholes." Here are some words of wisdom to be shared. Feel free to pencil in your own!

Beware of values gleaned through osmosis or your efforts will go up in smoke.

The process of assessing and articulating values is difficult work, and not quite as clear as other scientific and mechanical tasks. The health care organization, ministry department, and other personnel may sense certain values but may not be able to lay their hands on them. Values of course are oozing through the pores of all organizations and the persons within them. If left to ooze they will lose the power needed to keep the organization and hospital ministry alive. Values can, like smoke from the chimney of an old-fashioned fireplace, evaporate into thin air without providing essential heat or energy. This loss of energy will be less devastating if values are gathered and put to work.

Beware of inherited values or your burdens may be extra heavy.

Organizations, work groups, and individuals, tend to pass values down as a kind of inheritance. In ministry, the student chaplain learns about ministry, having perhaps been ministered to during childhood, youth, and young adult years. Since the average age of a person attending theological school is in the mid-forties today, chaplains are likely to have many years of hospital ministry values passed on to them. These values and their impact are probably brought into each new ministry setting.

As student and intern, the chaplain-intern inherits the values of teachers, supervisors, clinical settings, and persons and churches, who provide guidance and mentoring based on specific faith traditions. Early training experiences are crucial points of vulnerability from a value-defining perspective. While all these inherited values are quite helpful, and many are essential for the identity formation of a chaplain-intern, some are actually not very constructive and can be carried unconsciously throughout one's ministry with negative results.

Some values, like the weather, change daily.

Values are neither fixed nor constant. This is both good news and the impetus for identifying and harnessing values to the good of hospital ministry. Values are often paradoxical, and are certainly often not integrated within a person, group, or organization. Values are influenced by culture, resources, and beliefs. It is possible to ascertain that the multiplicity of acceptable values in today's world makes it crucial to reflect on values as a matter of course for each aspect of everyday living. It may be most helpful to continuously ask yourself or others, "What values are you reflecting right now, at this time?"

Some values are sacred and others may really be dinosaurs rather than epiphanies.

In the world of values, not all values are equal. Certainly, it is not possible to pay equal attention to the many and diverse values found in any given context during any given time. However, we are challenged to do our best. The notion of sacredness, of course, does not just apply to faith traditions, hospital ministries, or the chaplaincy discipline. Certainly, a few values rise to the very top of health care services and become fixed.

For example, a physician's oath, "to do no harm" is a sacred value, just as the mandate, "visit the sick," is a sacred Christian value. But some values such as, "this is the way we've always done it," or "we need to maintain the status-quo," may not be helpful in some situations. A word of caution: treat all sacred values with kid gloves.

To continue the dinosaur metaphor, we enjoy learning about the dinosaurs and treasure the remains found of these once-living creatures.

We even mourn their extinction. However, our energies need to be focused on saving those species that may be vulnerable today.

Being blind to values doesn't mean they don't exist.

According to Peter Senge and colleagues (Senge et al., 1994, p. 302), "When values are articulated but ignored, an important part of the shared vision effort is shut away." Values are observable in demonstrated behaviors and attitudes. Consciously deciding not to observe values at work in a given individual or context is perhaps understandable, but unwise. Conversely, seeing values at work can be enriching and empowering. In pastoral counseling and therapeutic enterprises we have a saying: "recognizing the giraffe in the room." By this we mean that something very powerful or large would be quite obvious if we would just look at it. It is a skill to notice when one's obvious value(s) are in place and/or activated. One is in denial whenever one thinks no values are involved in any of life's experiences or endeavors.

Values are not for the squeamish, nor are they for the silent.

Values are powerful thoughts, attitudes, concepts, and feelings. To access one's values and really face how they affect self and others, is to be engaged in the arena of energy and spirit. In this sense, values always come from the spiritual dimension, for they bring energy and spirit to meaning (vision) and they encourage meaningful purpose (mission) and mission-guided direction (goal-setting). To articulate values, or to determine how one will live-out one's values, is equivalent to taking a stand. Our values indicate who we are and what is important to us. It is impossible for values to be ignored or truly hidden. The best approach is to live and state your values, assess and change them as necessary, and boldly go about life and ministry as a value-laden enterprise.

Values tend to go for cover at the slightest perceived threat.

It seems to be a rule in life, as well as in relationships, that threat causes the fight-or-flight syndrome. In hospital ministry, staff, family, and patients tend to project, realistically or otherwise, their notions of what chaplains should value. At the same time, staff, family, and patients all have values that they may or may not be aware of at any given time. Some of these values may be perceived as unacceptable to a chaplain/clergy or to the idealized image that a person is trying to maintain. When a person feels vulnerable about his or her values, he or she usually tries to either reject the value (hide it and/or run from it), or reject the chaplain (fight). Recognizing and respecting values is essential to having, learning, and living with them.

Respect the individual's values while establishing shared values.

If we were all to live in separate universes, it might be possible to have static values that could be more constant and remain fixed for greater periods. However, this is not the real world. For those who value relationships, communities, and collaboration, dialogue is essential for values to live and to be spirit-filled.

A small story illustrates this point. My grandson Dylan was three years old and looking forward to eating some M&M's that he had received from his other grandmother. He had asked for those M&M's, and clearly valued them highly, certainly higher than he did the wonderful turkey sandwich and fries that his mother graciously made him for lunch. He waited all afternoon for those M&M's. After several hours, he once again requested and received the candies, and opened them with great enthusiasm. He ate one or two and looked at his mother for a moment. Then he walked over to her and asked if she would like to share. She did, and it was a wonderful thing.

It seems that in the world of common sense and experience, we learn early on to share, to respect one another, and to wonder if the thoughts, feelings, concepts, and beliefs we value are also valued by others. When this happens things work well, but when our thoughts, feelings, concepts, and beliefs are put down we are least likely to share them freely. Sharing is an essential part of teamwork, and is a value that many chaplains feel is crucial in hospital ministry. In fact, the sharing of very close, sometimes intimate thoughts, feelings, beliefs, and values, has always been at the heart of hospital ministry's role in healing.

You must use values or you might lose them.

It is a strange notion that one could lose values. However, radical changes tend to make it difficult to keep values current, relevant, and intact. This is particularly so in a time of decreasing space in what we fondly call our "global village," and in the pervasiveness of the connectedness that comes from a technically driven world that changes the way we think and live, seemingly, moment by moment. For hospital chaplains and pastors, one of the ways to lose values is to avoid mentioning them. Values are also lost when we don't plan for their use or when we defer to others for value definition.

Values are the path to meaning and purpose.

It is important to understand that spiritual care and hospital ministry are built on the foundations of value, meaning, purpose, and direction. This is a good thing, for it makes chaplains and clergy good candidates to support, encourage, and guide the efforts of individuals, departments, and hospitals as they go about their efforts to plan for and guide their endeavors in a health care facility.

VALUE AWARENESS EXERCISES

Some values stay with individuals, professions, and organizations, for very long periods of time. Indeed, many remain throughout the life of an individual, group, profession, or organization. Other values change. Either way, it is crucial for those engaged in hospital chaplaincy, pastoral and spiritual care, and ministry, to periodically review and reflect on the core values that are active in their ministry. These reflections will no doubt lead to increased awareness of values that are integrated in their ministry and to those that perhaps need further development. This kind of reflection will also bring to light ways in which one may have gone off course.

What follows are two value awareness exercises. The first exercise is designed to encourage this type of awareness and reflection at a personal level. The second is designed to open up the discussion of value-based ministry at departmental, parish, or organizational levels.

Exercise 1: "Personal Values I Bring to Hospital Ministry"

Instructions: Beginning with Exercise 4.1a, "Hospital Ministry and Theology Values," circle the number that best represents how you value each word or phrase and the importance you currently give it in your hospital ministry. The numbers range from 1 to 5, with 5 representing a strong, or higher, value for you; 1 represents an item that is of lower comparative value. The numbers in between represent values that are more or less strongly held. Circle the number that reflects your thinking or valuing of the word or phrase.

Example

When you read the word "collaboration," is it a value that you bring to hospital ministry and value very strongly? If so, circle 4 or 5 on the chart.

If collaboration is one of many values you bring to hospital ministry, but right now doesn't seem to be one of the most important, circle 3.

If collaboration is important, but not something you value very highly, you might circle a 2. Circle 1 if it really is not part of your set of values.

After you have completed Exercise 4.1a, continue with Exercise 4.1b, "Hospital Ministry and Health Care Values," and Exercise 4.1c, "Hospital Ministry and People Values." After you have made choices on each of the three charts, add the numbers circled and place your total point score at the bottom of each of the three tables.

EXERCISE 4.1a. Hospital Ministry and Theology Values

Salvation	1	2	3	4	5
Tradition	1	2	3	4	5
Church/Synagogue/ Mosque/Circle	1	2	3	4	5
Prayer	1	2	3	4	5
Sacrament	1	2	3	4	5
Worship	1	2	3	4	5
Call	1	2	3	4	5
Ministry	1	2	3	4	5
God/Christ	1	2	3	4	5
Ordination	1	2	3	4	5
Conversion	1	2	3	4	5
Miracles	1	2	3	4	5
Healing	1	2	3	4	5
Holy Days	1	2	3	4	5
Suffering	1	2	3	4	5
Presence	1	2	3	4	5
Spirituality	1	2	3	4	5

EXERCISE 4.1a *(continued)*

Belief	1	2	3	4	5
Holy Writings	1	2	3	4	5
Witness	1	2	3	4	5
Chapel	1	2	3	4	5
Presence	1	2	3	4	5

Total Score _____

EXERCISE 4.1b. Hospital Ministry and Health Care Values

Health	1	2	3	4	5
Illness	1	2	3	4	5
Wellness	1	2	3	4	5
Recovery	1	2	3	4	5
Pain management	1	2	3	4	5
Cure	1	2	3	4	5
Aftercare	1	2	3	4	5
Coping skills	1	2	3	4	5
Lifestyle changes	1	2	3	4	5
Patient care	1	2	3	4	5
Interventions	1	2	3	4	5
Medication	1	2	3	4	5
Diagnosis	1	2	3	4	5
Treatment plans	1	2	3	4	5
Mind, body, and spirit	1	2	3	4	5
Cost	1	2	3	4	5
Resources	1	2	3	4	5
Choices	1	2	3	4	5
Patient	1	2	3	4	5
Service delivery	1	2	3	4	5
Improvement	1	2	3	4	5
Satisfaction	1	2	3	4	5

Total Score _____

EXERCISE 4.1c. Hospital Ministry and People Values

People	1	2	3	4	5
Family	1	2	3	4	5
Connection	1	2	3	4	5
Home	1	2	3	4	5
Support	1	2	3	4	5
Diversity	1	2	3	4	5
Leadership	1	2	3	4	5
Collaboration	1	2	3	4	5
Teamwork	1	2	3	4	5
Counseling	1	2	3	4	5
Patient needs	1	2	3	4	5
Staff	1	2	3	4	5
Help	1	2	3	4	5
Serving	1	2	3	4	5
Changing	1	2	3	4	5
Individualized treatment	1	2	3	4	5
Caring	1	2	3	4	5
Respect	1	2	3	4	5
Hospitality	1	2	3	4	5
Communication	1	2	3	4	5
Patients first	1	2	3	4	5
Advocacy	1	2	3	4	5

Total Score _____

Scoring Your Values and Determining Your Hospital Ministry Profile

After you have completed Exercises 4.1a, b, and c, look at the profiles that follow. Remember that these exercises are awareness exercises and reflect only your responses to the words and phrases given. You may find that your value choices are high in all three areas, or you may find that your totals are a fraction more or less in any one given area. The idea is to increase your awareness of your values. Once you have looked at the three value profiles that follow, you may wish to continue with one or more of the additional value awareness exercises that I've included. You may want to journal about your thoughts and feelings. Feel free to write your value notes in the margins throughout this book. For those engaged in hospital ministry, and likewise for those who are setting up a hospital ministry program, you are encouraged to reflect on values already in place, as well as values driving your desires for hospital ministry.

A Theological Ministry Value Profile

It is understandable that those either engaged in or interested in hospital ministry are likely to rate theological words and phrases highly. There was a time when most chaplains were clergy and would likely value theology and religion highly in their ministries. In psychiatric settings, the earliest of hospital ministry personnel were parish clergy who visited patients in hospitals. When these persons became hired staff, they still focused on religious-based visitation and worship opportunities. In many general hospital settings of today, the hospital ministry program consists of visitation from area clergy. These clergy primarily visit persons of their own faith. Those who place a low value on theological words and phrases will likely have to set learning goals for themselves so they can minister to patients who have a need for more theologically based chaplains/clergy.

A Health Care Ministry Value Profile

It is highly unlikely that an experienced person would devalue health care values yet remain in health care settings. However, ambivalence about health care values can be just as strong as ambivalence about certain theological values. Persons who are low in the rating of health care values are encouraged to examine their ministry, their involvement, and their ministry's focus. Those who prefer to work closely with their hospital colleagues are encouraged to engage in transformative reflection and skill-building so they can move freely among the diverse values found in hospital settings.

A People Ministry Value Profile

It is quite unlikely that a person engaged in hospital ministry would be very low on the people value profile. However, if you are lowest on this profile it may be that you are at a crossroads in your ministry and could use a time of reflection, self-care, and perhaps a consultation about where you are and where you want to be. You may have had some traumatic experiences or just need a change of ministry setting. You may be stretching yourself too thin. Valuing people is crucial to hospital ministry. While it can be said that theological, health care, and people values are all essential to hospital ministry, it is impossible to be engaged in hospital ministry without focusing on people. If you are low in this area, take heart—there are lots of resources available.

Additional Ways to Increase Personal Value Awareness

Expanded brainstorming. You may wish to take the lists provided in the exercises, and brainstorm other words that come to you when thinking about hospital ministry, and thus increasing your awareness of your own values. When you brainstorm other words, do so without thinking positively or negatively about them. Just make a list. Spend two to five minutes writing down what comes to mind. After you have added your own words, see how they cluster together in themes. If you like, use other profiles than those previously discussed.

Circle preferences. You may be interested in noting preferences without clustering them into categories or profiles. In this case, circle the words you like most in the lists and add others as desired.

Value improvement exercise. After you have made your choices from the lists, go back and place a plus or minus next to each word or phrase. Use the plus to indicate that you feel you demonstrate that value well. Use the minuses to represent those words or phrases that you feel you would like either to develop further or have no interest in developing at this time. Choose five words or phrases that you would like to develop further, put them on a value development list. Prioritize these five values so that you can begin working on the first one or two. See also, Peter Senge and colleagues, in *The Fifth Discipline Fieldbook,* 1994, pp. 209-210.

Exercise 2: Value-Based Ministry at the Departmental or Parish Level

Instructions: Make copies of Exercise 4.2, "Value-Based Ministry at the Departmental or Parish Level." Gather together a hospital ministry work group.

Step 1.   Each person checks what is important to him or her from the list.

Step 2.   Each person adds value words or phrases to the list as desired.

Step 3. Members of the work group (department, program, team) dialogue with one another about the values each has chosen by focusing on the meaning of the value to them in their hospital ministry.

Step 4. The work group can then use a consensus process to prioritize values for their hospital ministry program/department. During this consensus-building process, the list is decreased to five or fewer as desired.

Note: It is crucial that everyone proceeds with the understanding that most items on the original and expanded list are likely to be valued by someone. Those which are not part of the group's final list of core values can still be valued by the group and by individuals.

THE DEVELOPMENT OF A HOSPITAL MINISTRY VISION STATEMENT

What Is a Vision?

A vision statement is "a clear image of what an organization could and should become if it is to realize its full potential" (Nolan, Goodstein, and Pfeiffer, 1993, p. 31). According to Nolan, Goodstein, and

EXERCISE 4.2. Value-Based Ministry at the Departmental or Parish Level

Availability	Services	Self-mastery	Empowerment
Relationships	Professional	Ethical	Wholeness
Mind/body/spirit	Recovery	Spirituality	Wellness
Timely	Pastoral care	Counseling	Biblically-based
Outcomes	Mission	Mastery	Reward and recognition
Action	Support	Collaboration	Leadership
Quality	Empathy	Presence	Skill-based
Compassion	Teamwork	Advocacy	Faith
Justice		Competencies	

Our Current Value-Based Ministry Priorities Are:
1.
2.
3.
4.
5.

Pfeiffer, a vision is a picture, a foundation, and an energy source. Furthermore, says, Peter Senge and colleagues (1994, p. 302), "a vision is an image of the desired future."

Vision As Picture

Both vision and picture are visual words describing what one wants to have or be in the future. One could use the word "map" to think of vision as where one would like to go or be. Vision speaks to the future and to possibility.

Vision As Foundation

Vision also speaks to grounding. In that sense it is the basis for any life or movement of person or organization.

Vision As Energy Source

Because vision dwells among the roots of past and present and moves and pulls us forward into the future, it can be described as an energetic process that is fueled by values and ignited by imagination. We are lost without vision. We may be able to climb a hill, but without vision we would not know what hill to climb and thus, would not know why it is important to climb the hill, having no plan or a reason for getting there.

Models of Vision-Based Hospital Ministry

While there are numerous visions of hospital ministry, the four following vision models are closer based on their prevalence in the field. They are presented as a means of encouraging chaplains and spiritual care providers to think about their own vision of hospital ministry. The four included are:

1. A single shared vision model
2. A responsible stewardship vision-setting model
3. A complementary visions model
4 A Babylon captivity vision model

A Single Shared Vision Model

In this model, vision and core values are established by upper management and are then shared with the rest of the organization. This is the prevalent model used by health care organizations trained in current theories of management and strategic planning. Once central leadership establishes core values and vision statements, it becomes middle managers' and staff's responsibility to be aware of and buy into the vision. This means that in an organization with 900 employees, approximately 15, or 1 percent, set the vision and core values for the whole organization. In this model, input from the rest of the organization is highly dependent on the interest and benevolence of the central leadership.

A Responsible Stewardship Vision-Setting Model

Peter Block, in *Stewardship, Choosing Service Over Self-Interest,* presents a stewardship model for organizational planning. He bases this model on the premise that individuals must use their personal values to create a vision for their work. Individual values and visions are shared with work groups who then dialogue about joint missions who then move on to specific jobs and tasks. Responsibility for vision remains with the individual, and no efforts are made to create a single organizational vision. Block goes further to declare that, "a vision created for others to live out is patriarchy in action. There is no ownership in endorsement or enrollment" (Block, 1993, p. 191). Furthermore, he says, "Each of us defining vision for our area of responsibility is how partnership is created" (Block, 1993, p. 192). It must be noted that this is not a common model in health care organizations today. However, it can be found in some hospital ministry departments.

Complementary Visions Model

A complementary vision model for hospital ministry may be found in situations where the overall organizational vision does not exactly match that of an individual department or service. It can also be found in situations where core values are not quite in sync. For example, such a model might be invoked in situations where the age-old debate about the differing values and focus of science and religion continues. When hospital ministry attempts to carry on its vision within a friendly setting with slightly differing values, there may be efforts on the part of the ministry and the organization to live with each other, and to even see complementary ways to use one another's values and services.

A Babylon Captivity Vision Model

Situations arise where the core values and visions of the hospital just don't seem to match those of the pastoral care department or ministry program. There are times when hospitals are uneasy, even a bit hostile, regarding certain faith traditions, chaplaincy, or ordained and clinically trained chaplaincy programs. This kind of hostility can vary in intensity. Chaplains who stick with such a situation often focus their ministry narrowly, try to be somewhat invisible, or focus on being a bit prophetic about moving the organization along, however slowly. In cases of subtle hostility between a hospital and its ministry, raising cultural awareness over time may work. In cases where the hospital is supportive, but individual units or persons have radically differing values and visions, it may help to dialogue undefensively about what each is trying to do. The Babylon captivity vision model is named in remembrance of the years that the Hebrew people spent in captivity in Babylon, the people who learned to sing and play their harps in a foreign land. Indeed, compared to parish ministry, hospital ministry is a bit of a foreign land!

Examples of Vision Statements
Along with Identified Core Values

Before writing a vision statement, it may be helpful to see examples of this type of statement. The following four are typical vision statements coming from various sources and focus on different forms of hospital ministry. In many cases it is difficult to choose one over another, but writing one's own statement, after seeing examples, can be quite energizing and certainly thought-provoking.

- Our vision is to be a catalyst for prophetic, transformational, and healing experiences. We value persons, equity and justice, and faith-centered living.
- Our Church's vision is to have a hospital ministry for members and friends. We value people, and believe that it is the church's place to provide spiritual resources to its flock.
- My vision is that I will fulfill my pastoral call to minister to the sick. I value my call, mission, stewardship, and Christian responsibility to those in need.
- Our vision is that there will be pastoral care available to all persons when they are hospitalized. What really matters to me/us in hospital ministry are the patients.

Exercise: Create a Vision Statement for Your Hospital Ministry

When writing a vision statement about your hospital ministry, remember to keep the statement short. You will probably write and rewrite this statement numerous times, so be prepared to consider your vision statement as provisionary until you develop one that really moves you and speaks to who you are and what you want to become.

A bit of advice: think grand! Every time you write a statement, think to yourself, "larger." This is crucial, for often clergy and pastoral personnel tend to minimize their visions as they go about the daily tasks of hospital ministry. It is easier to think about visiting patients and being a "presence" to people, than it is to wonder what could be. We always leave the "could be" type of thinking to the realm of the kingdom, miracles, and heaven.

Example of Grand Vision Thinking

A patient once helped me move from my practical, but perhaps confining, type of thinking into the realm of vocational vision. I remember this experience as a gift from a person who had numerous delusions, suffered from despair and depression, and was often quite hostile and filled with rage about having spent more than half a lifetime struggling with a major mental illness. The gift came in this form—the patient leaned back in a chair, looked me straight in the eye as peer and collaborator and stated, "I imagine you look forward to the time when you put yourself out of business." Now that's visionary thinking!

When developing your vision statement, ask yourself the following questions:

- Where do I (we) want to go or be in hospital ministry?
- What will it look like when I (we) get there?
- Am I thinking big enough?
- Is this a big picture way of looking at hospital ministry?
- What values and assumptions support this vision?

A Chaplain's Vision Statement with Core Values

My vision is _____

_____

_____

_____

This really matters to me because I value _____

_____

_____

_____

*Parish Clergy or Lay Minister's Pastoral Care
Vision Statement with Core Values*

My vision is _____

_____

_____

_____

This really matters to me because I value _____

_____

_____

_____

*Pastoral Care Departmental Vision Statement
with Core Values*

The Pastoral Care Department's vision is _____

_____

_____

_____

This really matters to us because we value _____

_____

_____

_____

*Parish Pastoral Care Hospital Ministry Vision Statement
with Core Values*

Our vision is _____

_____

_____

_____

This really matters to us because we value _____

_____

_____

_____

Turning Your Vision into a Mission Statement

What Is a Mission Statement?

A mission statement is "a brief statement . . . that identifies the basic business the organization is in" (Nolan et al., 1993, p. 135). A mission statement answers the question "What are we here to do together?" (Senge et al., 1994, p. 303). When developing a mission statement for hospital ministry, the group or individual must move from the question of "What is important to me/us?" (value) to "What is the future I/we would like to create?"(vision), and onward to asking "What is my/our purpose?"(mission). One way to look at the process of moving from value to vision to mission is to consider Timothy Nolan and colleagues' notion that "mission statements are actionable visions!" (Nolan et al., 1993, p. 46).

Models of Mission-Based Hospital Ministry

Just as there are multiple visions and values connected to hospital ministry, there are also multiple purposes. These purposes make up the mission of individuals and departments. Three typical mission models are:

- The Salvation and Witness Model
- The Visitation and Comfort Model
- The Holistic Healing Model

The Salvation and Witness Model

Some proponents of this model are likely to represent conservative faith traditions. The focus of ministry is clearly contained in the name—salvation and witness. In some cases this mission comes from the faith tradition of the chaplain/pastor and in other cases this mission corresponds with hospitalized persons' wishes.

Example. George entered a clinical pastoral education program while attending a conservative theological school, a requirement for graduating. George completed orientation in a general hospital and was assigned to the emergency room and to the oncology unit. He made several pastoral care visits and wrote his first verbatim from a visit with a middle-aged woman who was dying. This woman was not a Christian, nor did she wish to be one. She did appreciate his prayers up to the point where he insisted that she confess her sins and accept Christ as her savior. She got very angry and rang for the nurse. George was perplexed. He felt he was just doing his job. As he understood it, the woman was dying and his job was to witness to Christ and to help her accept Him so that she could be saved.

Another example. A chaplain-supervisor was called to visit a woman who insisted on seeing a chaplain. The chaplain-supervisor arrived and noted that the woman had pastoral care visits from two clinical pastoral education students in the past three days. However, he introduced himself and asked her if he could be of help. She was quite angry and asked, "Where are the Christian Chaplains? Aren't they supposed to be visiting patients and saving souls?" It turned out that one student had admitted she was a Unitarian. The other tried to listen and comfort the patient and said a prayer with her. However, neither student had checked on the woman's status with God in ways that the woman was used to hearing.

Another version of the salvation and witness model is one that relies on specific sacred words or sacraments as the basis of pastoral care. In these cases the representational role of the chaplain as belonging to a specific faith tradition is paramount to any contact. Salvation is still stressed in believing the Word and/or participating in the sacrament. In many cases this model is very welcome when used with patients who have similar beliefs and faith systems.

The Visitation and Comfort Model

Most chaplains, parish clergy, and spiritual care providers see visitation and comfort as their mission when visiting those hospitalized and their families. Those who use this model are usually good listeners and may use a variety of techniques to bring comfort. They may bring best wishes from congregations, devotional material and aids, and assistance in sorting out the thoughts and feelings that often accompany hospitalization and illness.

Example

Kim visited an elderly man who had just had bypass heart surgery. She asked how he was doing and he sighed heavily. When encouraged to go further, he shared with Kim his fear of going home and his concern for himself and his wife, who also had multiple health problems. He said he believed in God but this was too much! Kim stayed with him and let him talk for about twenty minutes. At that time he said he was grateful to her for listening to him. She asked if he would like to pray and they did so. Then she asked if there was anything else she could do for him. He told her that it would be nice if she could come back and visit the next day. Kim made a note to help him think of resources that he had to help him when he returned home. She decided to bring this up on the next visit.

The Holistic Healing Model

Persons who see the mission of their hospital ministry as focusing on holistic healing often are eclectic in their use of resources. They tend to work with the spiritual stresses and needs of each person on a one-to-one basis. They may state what their own traditions are but are careful to not force these traditions on others. In most cases they assess a patient's spiritual and religious beliefs and resources, and may determine that some of these beliefs and resources may not be currently helping the person in recovery. If this is the case, the chaplain may try to help the person sort out beliefs and practices to determine which are helpful, and which may not be helpful at the time. In some cases persons who see holistic healing as their ministry mission will draw upon a great variety of resources to help in the healing processes of individuals.

Many pastoral counselors and clinically trained chaplains are believers in holistic healing focuses. Often, this model works well with other disciplines and fits into the treatment planning processes in most hospital settings.

Example. Jean arrived at the psychiatric hospital very depressed and was experiencing some psychotic features. She belonged to a conservative Christian church and was hearing the voice of Satan. The chaplain was called in to support Jean and see if there were other ways to help her. She seemed so frightened. Working with Jean and the treatment team, the chaplain was able to gather a variety of resources and make them available to Jean and the team. The chaplain was able to support Jean's beliefs while helping her through hallucinogenic material that was part of the psychosis.

Examples of Hospital Ministry Mission Statements

Following are four examples of hospital ministry mission statements. Again, each one is of value depending on one's assumptions, values, and vision of hospital ministry. Mission, just like vision, does not remain fixed. While the thrust on one's ministry may change, grow, and develop, the refinement of how that happens often changes with time.

- The purpose/mission of my hospital ministry is to serve the spiritual needs of the persons who are hospitalized at this hospital.
- The purpose/mission of my hospital ministry is to develop a chaplaincy-based pastoral care department at this hospital.
- The purpose/mission of my hospital ministry focus is to visit persons from my parish who are hospitalized.
- The purpose/mission of our hospital ministry program is to set up a system for enhancing the services we provide to persons from our parish who are hospitalized.

Exercise: Create a Mission Statement for Hospital Ministry

When creating a mission statement, remember to keep it short. Mission statements that are long and involved often suffer from lack of focus, clarity, and lack the ability to serve as movement motivators. Complete as many mission statements as apply to you and your situation. Questions to ask yourself are: "What is my/our mission or purpose?" and/or "Why am I here?" Remember that mission statements are more specific than vision statements and grow out of vision and values.

A Chaplain's Mission Statement

The purpose/mission of my hospital ministry is to _____

_____

_____

_____

A Parish Clergy or Lay Minister's Pastoral Care Mission Statement

The purpose/mission of my hospital ministry is to _____

_____

_____

_____

A Hospital Ministry's Departmental Mission Statement

The purpose/mission of our/the department's hospital ministry is

_____

_____

_____

Parish Pastoral Care Hospital Ministry Mission Statement

The purpose/mission of our pastoral care/hospital ministry program is _____

_____

_____

_____

AREAS OF GROWING CONCERN

Hospital ministry is carried on in a specific context with a set of expectations and values consisting of a body of standards and traditions. Of course, there are variances due to the uniqueness of each hospital and its personnel. Today's chaplains must pay particular attention to several changing values that affect hospital ministry. These changing values are also thrust on hospitals as a whole, and no longer addressing them is simply no longer an option. Therefore, the following three areas are crucial to developing a mission and carrying out shared visions of pastoral care services:

- Diversity of spirituality, styles, and traditions
- Age-specific considerations
- Inclusivity concerns

Diversity

If there is such a thing as a "state-of-the-art" hospital ministry, that ministry must include the valuing of spiritual diversity. Regardless of the faith/spiritual tradition of chaplains, provision must be made to demonstrate respect and value of all persons. Services must include resources for varying faith traditions, respect and services for persons with no faith traditions, and the same for those with no identified set of beliefs. This means that a Catholic priest just for Catholics, a Protestant minister just for Protestants, and a Rabbi just for those of Jewish faith is no longer sufficient.

Example

When I began work at New Hampshire Hospital fifteen years ago, I taught new employees that 50 percent of patients were likely to be of Roman Catholic background; 50 percent were likely to identify themselves as Protestants; up to four persons at any given time identified themselves as Jewish; and once in a while there would be a person or two from a non–Judeo-Christian tradition. I was able to determine this by looking at the hospital's daily census that carried religious preferences upon admission. Now, when I do a freeze frame of religious preferences, I find up to 15 percent define their faith traditions as unknown or none. I am just as likely to be asked for Wicca resources as I am for spiritual care resources that are to contain "none of that religious stuff."

Hallmarks for respecting diversity when it comes to pastoral and spiritual care, do not stop at hospitality and respect for differences. Rather, it means the inclusion of equitable and just services for all persons. This change in values means that persons engaged in hospital ministry must be broadly and continuously educated to be highly resourceful in these areas.

Age-Specific Considerations

Age-specific considerations are more than the development of clinical competencies and professional privileging processes. The movement toward developing skills for differing age groups is also based on a valuing of persons at different points in their lives. Children are valued as children, not as little adults, nor are they only valued as dependents, but as individuals with needs that must be valued in and of themselves. The same would be true of adults and of elder adults. The point to be made, in terms of values and hospital ministry, is that increased knowledge and length of life bring to the forefront of our ministry mission the need to be able to relate resourcefully to persons of varying ages because we value them.

Example

Twenty years ago, persons studying for the ministry in New England had to select clinical training sites for an approved training program in clinical pastoral education. The sites of highest value and desirability were general hospital sites. Much lower, but still next on the list of desirable sites, were psychiatric hospitals. Seldom did anyone have on their list the desire to work with "the kiddies" or with old people. Devaluing of elders and children is no longer acceptable. Values have changed and hospital ministry programs can no longer avoid missions that demonstrate the value of all.

Inclusivity

While it might be said that the value of inclusivity is implicit in the preceding sections, issues of diversity and age are mentioned separately because of their value and ability to motivate visions of what hospital ministry could and should be. Inclusivity is also based on value, vision, and mission. This value is not intended to mean that hospital ministry should be all things to all people. Rather, hospital ministry is a service and a place for all to be. Categories of inclusivity include: religious preference, types of illness, gender, ethnicity, culture differences, age, and sexual orientation.

PUTTING VISION AND MISSION INTO PRACTICE

Incorporating Vision and Mission into Hospital Policy, Scope of Practice Statements, Goal Setting, and Job Descriptions

Having developed vision and mission statements, the task becomes one of filling in that picture. One realizes their picture of hospital ministry first by defining what is called a "Hospital Ministry Scope of Practice." This scope of practice indicates what one's ministry will be. Next, standards or policies that need to be in place are identified. Job descriptions are written and revised. Finally, plans for short and long term goals are established along with ways in which these goals will be achieved.

Even as this last paragraph was being written, I knew some of my former colleagues and mentors who would be "turning in their graves" over all this "paper" work. Many chaplains have gotten out of the field because they could not get over having to do personal errands on their own time, or sitting in departmental meetings instead of being out there with the people. Times have indeed changed from when the chaplain could wander in, out, about, and around. Perhaps the services are no better now, but they are more explicit and more accountable to others!

To assist in the task of incorporating vision and mission into hospital policy, scope of practice, goal setting, and job descriptions, more information is located in the Appendix. There one will find:

- A sample copy of the department of pastoral services policy statement (Appendix D)
- A sample Scope of Practice Statement with achievement and goals identified (Appendix E)
- Sample job descriptions (Appendixes F, G, H)
- A sample service brochure (Appendix I)

The Development of Parish-Based Mission and Scope of Practice Statements for Churches

It is possible to use the exercises in this chapter, as well as other material in this book, to develop parish programs focused on hospital ministry. While parish clergy or lay visitors may not see themselves as "chaplains" while engaged in hospital ministry, it would be helpful to take to heart many of the skills and practices suggested in this book. In some cases, clinically trained chaplains supervise and support clergy in their pastoral care and hospital ministry endeavors. This approach is sometimes taken a step further when a church decides to treat its hospital ministry program with the same kind of intentionality that it treats its other programs.

Where Does Your Ministry Fit?

Are you starting from scratch? Are you revising vision and mission statements that are tired, out of date, and no longer motivating? Do you have parts and pieces and need to put it all together? Don't be discouraged. Recently I asked two colleagues to read a draft of this book. I wanted their input while I was in the process of writing so I could take advantage of any wisdom they might have to offer. One person, a twenty-two-year veteran in chaplaincy and an educator, declared with some enthusiasm, "That chapter on developing a vision and a mission for hospital ministry was challenging and very helpful. I have never seen such a chapter included in a book on hospital ministry. Some of the steps that are good for us are not always easy to learn!"

Chapter 5

Integrating Professional Needs into the Practice of Hospital Ministry

A gift is like a seed; it is not an impressive thing. It is what can grow from the seed that is impressive. If we wait until our seed becomes a tree before we offer it, we will wait and wait, and the seed will die from lack of planting in the warm, moist earth. The miracle is not just the gift; the miracle is in the offering, for if we do not offer, who will? (Muller, 1996, p. 242)

Deanna Bellandi writes about the chaplain's life, "While some aspects of the chaplain's world remain unchanged, time has altered others. The 21st century chaplain must deal with increasing religious and ethnic diversity. Chaplains, too, have changed, with many more lay people tending to the spiritual needs of patients" (2000, p. 14). Bellandi quotes a Catholic priest from Cook County Hospital in Chicago, Reverend John Pennington, who says of the work he does as chaplain, "At their most vulnerable moment, you can bring some beauty into people's lives and make it a prayerful experience" (Bellandi, 2000, p. 16).

Few professions remain static in their scope and practice. In this respect chaplaincy and hospital ministry are no different from other professions. While the role of the chaplain and the practice of hospital ministry would be recognizable in the twenty-first century, just as it was recognizable 150 years ago, some things have changed. For one thing, the clinical training of chaplains has become a large skill-based venture that adds richness to growing academic offerings. Additionally, the research around chaplaincy, its focus, and outcomes has contributed greatly to standards and services, especially over the last twenty years. If anything, the field of hospital ministry has grown form infancy to maturity as we move into the twenty-first century.

In this chapter, a holistic model is used to provide an integrative look at some of the professional needs of hospital ministry personnel. Throughout the chapter, the reader will find first-person experiences of first-time students, mature clergy, supervisors, and chaplains. In all cases, specific experiences, where quoted, are meant to be anonymous and are used with permission. These quotes may be adapted with portions omitted for the purpose of focusing on the area at hand. Vignettes and experiences not quoted are composite material gathered together by the author and represent no one person or situation.

A STUDENT'S EXPERIENCE

Beginning clinical pastoral education is intimidating as all beginnings are difficult for me. It was particularly hard to hear so much enthusiasm from hospital staff about being "Christian," and being of service under that title. I cringe when I hear this label because it does not represent inclusive values to me and I do not wish to be identified with any exclusive group. Still, my supervisor kept returning to the theme of respect for others' traditions, helping me to feel less like an alien.

Ministering to individuals in crisis, coping with life threatening medical procedures, facing death and dying will be extremely challenging despite my life experience. I am praying for the humility and willingness to follow God's will for me. I pray for the presence and calm to be with people in suffering and pain, to find words to console and care. "Make me an instrument of thy peace . . ."

I am afraid of my humanness, my ability to enter into pain and suffering with others. I shed tears with others without censure when I am so moved. Is this OK? I know too well the pain of loss and the fear of facing the unknown. I join well. This is a new role, thus new boundaries accompanying this new profession—when are tears acceptable? I cannot imagine being present when news of someone's death is told to the family or loved ones without entering into a sacred sharing that includes tears. Other hospital personnel who witness the end of life for a dear patient, must have similar experiences so I will learn from them. This is only week one.

WHAT DOES A PERSON NEW
TO HOSPITAL MINISTRY NEED?

In the middle of a clinical pastoral education unit at Beverly Hospital (7-2000), Beverly, Massachusetts, students were asked to reflect on the question, "What does a person new to hospital ministry need?" It was hoped that these students would identify needs that could then be extrapolated for entry-level clergy. While the students' responses were somewhat bound to clinical issues often found with first unit clinical pastoral education studies, they nevertheless, provide a beginner's look at the hospital system and the role of those engaged in hospital ministry.

Responses to this inquiry were given verbally in a brainstorming format, then grouped according to a model that identifies the "five dimensions of the person": Physical, Emotional, Social, Intellectual, and Spiritual (Beck, Rawlins, and Williams, 1998, p. 174). Once sorted into these five categories, the responses were examined to try to understand which entry-level needs were being identified. In some cases a direct correspondence was apparent between student responses and specific identifiable entry-level needs. A handful of responses that seemed to relate only to the training program were omitted.

After the student's brainstorming session, chaplain Joan Rossi and supervisor, Reverend John C. Pearson, worked together to devise a list of what they thought newcomers to hospital ministry needed to know. This list was also grouped according to the same holistic model and sorted accordingly.

What follows is a review of the professional needs of persons engaged in hospital ministry from the perspectives of persons in very formative stages, to those engaged in this vocation for some twenty-two years.

NEEDS OF PERSONS ENGAGED
IN HOSPITAL MINISTRY

About the Holistic Dimensions of Personhood

For at least a dozen years, the pastoral services department at New Hampshire Hospital in Concord has been teaching about holistic dimensions of personhood as put forth by Cornelia Kelly Beck, Ruth Parmelee Rawlins, and Sophronia R. Williams in their book, *Mental*

Health-Psychiatric Nursing: A Holistic Life-Cycle Approach (1988). This model is based on the assumption that "Each person is considered as a whole with many factors contributing to health and illness" (p. 161). Furthermore, according to these authors, the "Five major concepts are generally accepted premises of holistic health care philosophy. First, each person is multidimensional; one's physical, emotional, intellectual, social, and spiritual dimensions are in constant interaction with each other" (p. 182).

It is quite helpful to take the holistic model of personhood, as described by Beck, Rawlins, and Williams, and apply it to the needs of persons engaged in hospital ministry. When this application is made, taking the input of students and chaplains into consideration, the results become very practical and demonstrate the universality of certain needs and issues in hospital ministry in general. To see how these needs are integrated into a model for the professional practice of hospital ministry, see Figure 5.1. After reviewing this chart and the elaborations that follow, one is encouraged to identify his or her own professional ministry needs using the blank chart provided in Appendix J. Directions for this process will be included at the end of this chapter.

Physical Needs

The area of physical needs for persons entering hospital ministry was underreported in the student brainstorming activity at Beverly Hospital. The two areas mentioned were "stamina" and "space." The students were surely thinking of the intensity of a first unit of clinical pastoral education, and specifically about their reflections on a group room for their clinical work together. But, those working in the mind, body, and spirit worldview prevalent today know how crucial it is to identify the physical needs of all people, including chaplains and pastoral care personnel. Some of these physical needs include health, space, presence, stamina, stress management, and the setting and understanding of physical boundaries of self and others.

Physical Health

A call to ministry, and the pursuit of experiences, training, and/or ordination in preparation for chaplaincy, does not necessarily involve passing a physical examination. However, part of the orientation of a new hospital employee does usually require a physical exam and some regular tests that are the same, regardless of one's status as an employee. This seems natural to most hospital staff, and they greet the requirements nonchalantly. Clergy/chaplains, however, are often surprised and occasionally annoyed to find that they are not exempt from this requirement. In addition, changes in health status of employees,

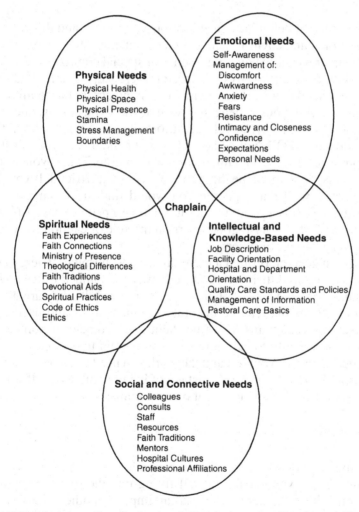

FIGURE 5.1. Integrating Professional Needs into the Practice of Hospital Ministry

including chaplains, are noted for their possible impact on patient health and care. Also of great import to hospital ministry staff is the training and self-protective procedures used by all employees to ensure physical safety and infection control throughout the hospital.

Physical Space (Physical Environment and Milieu)

Every human being has a need for physical space and this need is both personal and environmental. At a personal level, it is crucial for a chaplain or pastor to have some sense of special comfort or discomfort. To determine this physical space preference, ask a trusted colleague or friend to experiment with you. Stand across the room from one another. Ask your colleague to walk toward you slowly, one step at a time. As soon as you feel uncomfortable place your hand in the air to indicate STOP. Notice how close the person is to you. That is your preferred space when interacting with people. That is your comfort zone. Now do the same thing for your colleague/friend. If you did this exercise with many people you would find much variation in comfort zones. It is a good rule of thumb to give people space, at least three to six feet. It is also good to err on the side of caution for yourself and the benefit of others.

Space, in general, is often a premium in most hospitals. Clergy and chaplains may find themselves tucked away in cramped offices with minimum light and air circulation. In other hospitals, they are given nice airy offices that can be decorated to their tastes and needs. In some settings, chaplains may find themselves somewhat homeless, with no space really to call home. It is important to advocate for an identified space for yourself and the work you need to do on behalf of the hospital. Do not make the mistake of being humble or self-effacing to your own detriment or that of your ministry.

Physical Presence on Site

A student reflects: "My identity formation as a chaplain is progressing. I am experiencing myself fitting into the role as chaplain with grace. It's my presence that has an impact on others. I also feel that at times I can rise to the idea that I may be the answer to someone's prayers as I enter a patient's room."

It does not take long before a chaplain learns that presence is more than just a spiritual term. Indeed, presence is actually a very physical and incarnational need to be in contact with one another for chaplains, patients, family, and staff. Physical presence is something many persons in hospital ministry have difficulty with, both in terms of availability and the physical closeness of hundreds or thousands of persons working and receiving services in a hospital setting.

Hospital chaplains need to find physical space to handle the demands of providing physical presence in the hospital setting. They are not as free as parish clergy to set their work schedule. This is a blessing if you are a person who likes a scheduled and fairly predictable work week, or if you work in a hospital where you are not the only one providing coverage. However, it often comes as a surprise to new chaplains that their workday is set and they must work the whole day. The need to be physically present throughout the workday can be quite an adjustment.

Example. A chaplain who worked in a hospital during the 1960s, when one could live on the hospital campus and come and go reasonably flexibly, found that the work schedule ethic had changed in the mid-1990s. During these latter times, the chaplain had to write in the hour and minute of arrival and the hour and minute of departure. During his exit interview one year later, the chaplain complained about having to do his errands on his own time! He had apparently struggled privately over the "presence" issue.

In addition, parish clergy often find that there have been changes in their ability to engage in hospital ministry. Many parish clergy still expect to be able to come and go at will, by prerogative of their status as clergy. More frequently, clergy now find that they may be limited to the allotted visiting hours for the hospital, with no deference to their vocation. These changes in practice and philosophy make it essential that parish clergy and chaplains know the parameters of their physical presence according to current hospital regulations and/or the terms of their employment.

Stamina

Hospital ministry requires a certain type of energy that must be sustained in what can be challenging situations. Physical stamina, or healthiness, is crucial for a chaplain who needs to be able to move around well and perform emotionally challenging work. In this sense, physical self-care can often be forgotten or take second place, a problem shared with all caregivers. Of course stamina is quite related to physical, spiritual, emotional, social, and intellectual factors. Extra energy is always required to learn new things, to experience challenging events, and to empathize with persons in need.

Stress Management

A student reflects on a growing reliance on stressful events of a first unit clinical experience by declaring, "My last 'on call' was very quiet. I realized that I wanted the challenge of the more stressful events. I am able to assess the time I need to unwind after really being there fore people. My most rewarding experiences are those that take the most out of me."

It is quite possible to become physically addicted to putting oneself in situations that are highly challenging. It is also possible that some people are attracted to hospital ministry because of its perceived intensity and abundance of critical care situations. However, the results of continuous exposure to stressful situations, even those that are chosen, will eventually lead to complications for the health care provider. Taken to the extreme, poor stress management leads to professional burnout.

There are abundant resources for stress management. Most hospital settings have wellness activities and resources for physical exercise in particular. At the professional level, knowledge about stress management and the modeling of healthy life choices is crucial to providing pastoral care services.

Boundaries

The teaching and learning of professional boundaries is integral to the policies and standards of all hospitals. These professional boundaries are to be adhered to by all employees, including clergy and chaplains. When chaplains and/or clergy get into difficulties with physical boundaries in the hospital setting, they frequently are not paying attention to one of the following:

- Refraining from touching people
- Refraining from entering rooms when not wanted or when there is a universal precaution sign
- Refraining from entering rooms where delicate personal interventions or activities may be taking place
- Refraining from checking when doors are closed partially or fully or curtains drawn
- Refraining from long, tiring, and intrusive visits
- Refraining from touching or using any item in the patient's room without knowledge, permission, or clinical privileging

Emotional Needs and Feelings

In the brainstorming activity described at the beginning of this chapter, the students reflected on their feelings of awkwardness, discomfort, anxiety, and fear. They thought that persons new to hospital ministry might feel likewise. In this case, students were anxious and fearful about making visits, about silence, and about responding to emergencies. Of course, similar feelings are likely to be felt by persons in new hospital positions, particularly the first hospital visit after a person has finished training.

Established chaplains and chaplain supervisors were more aware of their reactions to a person in pain. These reactions were likely to be emotional, physical, and spiritual, and often lead to personal grief reactions by the professional caregiver. Established chaplains and chaplain supervisors were also more aware of their tendencies, and the tendencies of students, to avoid doing the very thing they were trained to do and are good at doing. This emotional resistance often comes in the form of avoiding visitation.

Self-Awareness

Toward the end of a first clinical unit a student writes, "I'm starting to feel like I don't have a self because I'm being pulled in so many directions at once. But my worry is that I am taking on a new profession that will leave me with less *self* than I've ever had. I'm tired. I keep crying and I just want to stop."

Midway through a first clinical unit, another student reflects on the issue of self-awareness: "I have learned that it is important to have a good sense of my self when I enter a pastoral situation. If I don't feel confident in being there, it will be easy for me to feel inadequate and get pushed around by the patient and/or the family's needs."

Self-awareness grows and develops throughout the professional lifespan. Also, it is tied not only to the concept we have of ourselves, but also to the feelings we attach to our understandings of self. In addition, self-awareness has an interpersonal component consisting of how we see ourselves in relation to others. At the mature level of ministry, one is able to know oneself reasonably well, and be a flexible self in relation to others. From this perspective, self-awareness is a professional tool used to the benefit of self and of others.

Management of Discomfort

There are many occasions when hospital ministry is uncomfortable. Certainly patients and their families are often uncomfortable too. The task of ministering to persons in varying intensities of discomfort, pain, and trauma is a challenging task. For a person new to this type of ministry, there are likely to be many situations that cause feelings of discomfort. However, this discomfort does not necessarily go away with time. At the mature level of professional growth, discomfort is a feeling that can be a sign or indicator of valuable knowledge about self or other people and situations.

According to one chaplain-educator, "I often tell students, 'If I ever stop feeling anxious/uncomfortable while visiting a patient, I will stop doing this work.' I will have become callous and blasé and unhelpful."

Awareness of Feelings of Awkwardness

Awkwardness is a form of discomfort, although it may have more of a self-judging component that the feeling of discomfort may not have. The students surveyed felt awkward, particularly with regard to the issue of silence in relational settings. They were also self-conscious about just about everything they did, were asked to do, or did not do. Such is the predicament of adult learners in new situations where they have not mastered a new skill. Time, practice, and growth in professional identity will ease these feelings in some, but not all, situations. In some cases, awkwardness on the chaplain's part constitutes a firm grasp on the reality of the hospital and health care realm, where the medical model is firmly embraced, and where the spiritual care model may or may not be so entrenched in the culture.

Management of Anxiety

Anxiety is likely to be a common and natural response to the newness of a position and may reflect real, as well as imagined, expectations. The students who engaged in the brainstorming session were particularly anxious about crisis situations.

One student from another clinical unit could name the anxiety through the use of only one word: overwhelming. In a first unit of clinical training during the first week of hospital ministry a student wrote, "The first day I was overwhelmed. The second day I was still overwhelmed, but realized that I would not remember many things until I actually did them. The third day I was still overwhelmed, but not totally. At the close of these three days I have accomplished becoming less overwhelmed."

Anxiety, as with all other feelings mentioned here, is not limited to the professional capacities of chaplains and clergy. The reason for this prevalence of anxiety has to do with the depth of experiences of professionals relative to the needs of those hospitalized, and the need for professional persons to dig deeper into themselves in order to provide ways to be of service to these individuals. What works in one situation may or may not work in others. While standards exist for hospital ministry, these standards are always subject to both human and divine hands. Even experienced pastors find new settings and experiences unsettling.

Example

An experienced parish pastor began a fifth clinical training unit with the following comments: "Starting out a new venture, or acquainting myself with a new site, contributed to a definite rise in anxiety over the past week to ten days. Finding my way around the hallways . . . to the various meeting rooms was quite disorienting." Later on, a chaplain-intern writes, "At this time, I simply need a general sense of location and orientation to feel comfortable and prepared for pastoral care visits; I'm nearly there."

Management of Fears

Students typically feared doing new things and facing the realities found in a hospital setting. The same thing applies to everyone, to one degree or another. Again, feelings like anxiety, awkwardness, and discomfort may abate with time and experience, but are unlikely to disappear entirely.

One student reflects insightfully, "I came to understand that I was so focused on joining and pastoral presence that I completely missed out on learning how to assess and respond to the needs of the patient. I was captured by my own fear of the situation."

Another chaplain, engaged in ministry in a psychiatric setting, found that it took almost fifteen years to get over the fear of offending a patient by asking him or her to leave a therapy group. The patient's anger and aggressiveness were thinly held in check when the chaplain knew the group was not helpful to the patient who was bringing down the rest of the group and causing chest pains for the chaplain-therapist. Some fears are imagined; others are quite reasonable. Attention should be paid to all fears when they arise. Genuine and persistent fears should be taken to a colleague for a professional consult and/or to a therapist or other resource.

Management of Resistance

A student reflects early on in a clinical training unit, "Doing this work is like walking into the mouth of the dragon. This is the most frightening work I have ever done. I have more than a passing acquaintance with death, but this work is like standing on the precipice looking at this grim reality about human existence. When I face going on call, like today, I feel the most incredible dread! I don't want to do this, or feel this. I don't want to stand out here on this cliff."

Resistance is included under emotional needs and feelings as it is usually a signal that a strong feeling or group of feelings have just become energized. Questions to ask when resistance is noted are:

- What am I resisting?
- What do I feel about that which I am resisting?
- What resources can I use to work through this resistance?
- If I cannot or do not want to work through the resistance, what does that mean for me and my ministry?
- Is it possible that the resistance I am feeling has come to me through the patient, family, or staff person? Is it their issues I am responding to or avoiding?

Feelings of Intimacy and Closeness

It is not a surprise that none of the students verbally noted the need for chaplains to come to grips with feelings of closeness and intimacy. Those surveyed through their written material were likely to note states of feelings, but did not explore feelings of intimacy and closeness. However, these feelings are just as prevalent as those of fear and anxiety.

In truth, it is not possible to engage in ministry without developing feelings of closeness without experiencing intimacy with persons. The important thing for a professional to know is that these feelings are natural, but expressing them is inappropriate, other than in the most professional sense. When you notice that you feel especially close to a person, it is always a good idea to get a quick consult, no matter how many years you have been in the ministry field. If any feelings of intimacy arise, it would be wise perhaps, to also check in with a therapist or other trusted and nonbiased professional. When feelings of intimacy and extra closeness come into question, do nothing with the patient, family, or other staff until you consult with a colleague.

Basic Confidence

A student reflects on the first week of clinical experience: "I am not sure what will make me feel comfortable on the units. I think the first steps in that direction will be getting to know the managers and plunging into the work."

Feelings of confidence come from management of uncomfortable feelings and increased pleasurable feelings. Feelings of confidence can also come from increased knowledge, practice, and skill building. In uncomfortable situations, a feeling of knowing what to do can make a situation tolerable, even when the situation is not pleasurable. With time and practice come feelings of confidence that stem from realistic understandings of one's role and tasks, and the ability to be creative about meeting the needs of hospitalized persons, their families and staff.

Expectations

A student writes in the second month of an extended first clinical unit, "I have been adrift in a sea of insecurity. Everything is new and there are no easy answers to any of the challenges that constantly pour forth. Each interaction with patients, clients, residents, and staff is a source of tension. This is difficult to admit. I have always been able to keep on going and 'do it all,' and guess what? I can't. On one level, it makes me feel sad and somewhat defeated. On another, it feels like a little bit of a burden is lifted because maybe it's ok to say 'no' to some things. I have a long way to go before I will be truly comfortable letting go however, I know I have to do so."

Expectations, whether internal or external, are often the source of multiple feelings. The feelings we have about these expectations are the reason this area is listed under emotional needs of professional persons. Emotionally, the difference between a professional and a student has much to do with how he or she manages internal and external expectations, and the ensuing feelings arising from these expectations. These will always be expectations. How we choose to handle these expectations includes the feelings we have about them.

Personal Needs

Professional persons have personal needs that may or may not be related to their vocation. One of the hardest things about being a chaplain is knowing how to separate personal needs from those of others. One of these is the need to have one's own feelings even if it is not helpful nor appropriate to express them. Some of these feelings and needs will be difficult for a chaplain to face, particularly in the novice years. Others will perhaps unconsciously bubble up in later years when one is stressed or in a life stage developmental phase.

Social and Connective Needs

The typical social or connection/networking needs of persons in hospital ministry are crucial for the development and establishment of professional identity and for the delivery of services. The students surveyed confirmed this through their positive feedback regarding the helpfulness of professionals who came into their programs. These same students recorded, time and again, incidents of contact with other professionals. They focused primarily on what was helpful and what was not helpful. In a clinical training program, much attention is often spent on connections with other staff. Clearly this relational need is crucial to students in their learning and identity formation.

Making connections and networking are also essential needs for professional chaplains and clergy working in hospital settings. However, establishing and nurturing such connections is an ongoing challenge. Frequent changes in personnel make staying up to date on who is who difficult. The nature of chaplaincy work in a medical setting, and the smallness of pastoral care departments, create further networking challenges. Whereas most hospital departments have numerous employees, most pastoral care departments consist of only one or two chaplains.

Regardless of the size of a pastoral care department, it is important to the professional growth and development of the chaplain or clergy/spiritual care provider to focus on the issues of joining and networking with other professionals within and outside of their discipline. Several networking areas to highlight would be meeting with colleagues, setting up of supportive and consultative relationships, and looking for general resources and mentoring opportunities.

Relating to Other Clergy and In-House Colleagues
in Pastoral Care

The nature of most pastoral care departments makes teamwork and harmony of purpose and function essential in the delivery of quality services. The same closeness is essential for supportive purposes. Chaplains who have difficulty with this closeness within the pastoral care profession are likely to become either isolated and somewhat of a lone ranger, or they are likely to begin turning to other staff for connective needs. While it is essential to connect well with staff and colleagues from all disciplines, it is also essential to remember that the chaplain, like the parish pastor, is always the chaplain. This means that the chaplain is the minister/priest/rabbi or care provider for staff, families, patients, and visitors. The chaplain is never off duty while in the hospital setting, except when in the presence of colleagues within the department.

Establishing a Support Base for Processing and Consulting

Standards of professional practice require that every professional person have a knowledgeable consultant available for the processing of professional material that he or she cannot process alone. The stress here is on the importance of the consult occurring with a "knowledgeable" person. If a chaplain is the sole person of his or her vocation in the hospital setting, then it is not sufficient to consult solely with persons from other disciplines. In some cases, it may be essential to covenant with persons from other hospital settings for consultative needs. These consultations do not have to be rigid as to time, format or frequency. Nor are consultations with persons in hospital ministry to be considered in lieu of consults with persons in other disciplines within the hospital setting.

Connecting with Hospital Staff

It is often said that it takes from six months to a year for an individual to get up to speed in a new job. In the case of hospital ministry, that time can be as long as several years. It is important to approach this task in manageable ways. One might get to know one person at a time, or, one might focus a bit more on persons in a single department such as nursing, social services, or psychology. One might also try to spend time in individual treatment teams where patients have either requested or are receiving pastoral care services. Connections are essential and are built over time. It is helpful to remember the possibility that staff know about you before you feel you know anything about them.

Setting Up Specialized Resources

Today's hospital chaplains are trained to relate to persons regardless of their faith traditions. However, one chaplain cannot provide services needed for each and every patient, staff, or family member who requires them. Getting to know what services are available throughout the hospital is essential. When working with staff, it is important to know what other resources are available. For example, there may be an employee assistance program available to staff. There may be counselors in the larger community available and willing to take referrals. The hospital may have a complaint investigator or an ombudsman available for patients with treatment concerns. It is quite common for the chaplain to be in a position of helping people get connected with resources. To be helpful in making these connections, the chaplain has to build up a well of resources that he or she can have readily at hand. Sometimes the greatest resource will be to know people who know about available resources.

Networking with Persons from a Variety of Faith Traditions

It seems that the nature and variety of faith traditions and spiritual care needs are constantly growing. Certainly there is a growing complexity of beliefs and practices. In-house chaplains cannot possibly meet all needs, although they can cover most services required. In cases requiring specialized services, contacts need to be in place. General hospital settings have an easier time at meeting this need than psychiatric hospitals. The stigma and unknown factors about mental illness make it a strenuous task to find people who are willing to be available for emergency services. Nevertheless, such resources are essential to the whole hospital ministry program.

Finding Mentors

Mentors are important resources throughout the professional life-span. During the formation and training process, mentors are often teachers and supervisors. Informally, they may also be persons from other disciplines, or chaplains who are not directly involved in the training program. However, the role and importance of the mentor does not end with academic, field, or clinical training. If anything, the mentor is crucial throughout one's ministry. Typical times for mentoring include the formative days on a new job; when one has been in hospital ministry over seven years; times when one has been in a place for twelve years or more; and times when one is considering leaving hospital ministry for retirement or to move into something else. It is helpful to think of mentors as those who have successfully bridged the stage or process you are beginning to try to bridge. Mentors can be consciously chosen or can be intuitively found. Mentors do not have to be from one's specific discipline.

Professional Affiliations

Numerous professional affiliations are available to chaplains. It is important to find one that meets your needs. These affiliations do not need to be large, established organizations; although belonging to such groups is a good idea. Local affiliations can be helpful. Some states have grass roots chaplaincy groups that are quite successful. If you are not connected with a chaplaincy group, or want to find out about other resources, it is helpful to ask around and find out what groups chaplains in your area find helpful. Recognized professional organizations to which chaplains may belong include:

- The Association of Clinical Pastoral Education
- The Association of Professional Chaplains
- The National Association of Catholic Chaplains
- The American Association of Pastoral Counselors

Making Connections with a Hospital's Culture

Every organization has its own established values, behaviors and patterns. "These recurring patterns of behavior are what many call the culture of the organization" (Wheatley, 1999, p. 128). By observing how persons within the organization relate to one another, it is possible to discover what the predominant culture is and what values are espoused. These behaviors and values shape the organization and help hospital ministry personnel know how their work will be received within the organization as a whole. There will be times when hospital ministry has a marginal place and value, and there will be times and settings where hospital ministry is just as valued as any other hospital service. Knowing how to relate to the hospital's culture is as essential as knowing how to relate to each individual within his or her context.

Intellectual and Knowledge-Based Needs

Job Description

Whether student or chaplain, it is essential to know what is expected in any given situation. Those who have had clinical pastoral education experiences presumably know some of the expectations of being a chaplain. However, the role of student is quite different from that of professional chaplain. Thus, it is not always easy for an individual to move into the professional role of chaplain. This makes it crucial for the new chaplain to look closely at job descriptions. Those who are experienced in hospital ministry know to expect and ask for a job description.

Unfortunately, many clergy do not have clear job descriptions nor are such descriptions necessarily the basis of evaluation of their job performance. Thus, when parish clergy move into the hospital setting they may be unprepared for the ways in which hospital personnel are evaluated. In hospital ministry, the connection between job description and yearly evaluation is the basis of standard personnel processes.

For those who wonder about job descriptions, samples may be found in the appendixes. These samples are provided for purposes of comparison and to help persons and institutions develop their own job descriptions. Sample job descriptions include two supervisory role descriptions and one entry-level job description currently in use at New Hampshire Hospital in Concord (see Appendixes F, G, and H).

Facility Orientation

Simple things such as the provision of a map, a floor plan, and a tour of the facility should be part of the orientation every new employee needs. Since chaplains will need to be able to respond to pastoral care calls from the very beginning, it is a good idea to take the time to learn what is where in the facility. Should your hospital be complex, and/or spread out, the rule of thumb for most chaplains is to ask a secretary, or make a quick call to the switchboard. When you go to specific areas of the hospital make sure to check for signs and directions letting you know whether you can enter an area or a specific patient's room. You should learn about the programs and rules of differing units and receive safety and infection control training before going to any patient units. If you do not get this training (chaplains are sometimes overlooked) take the initiative and ask for it, for your protection and for the protection of others.

Hospital and Department Orientation

Every hospital has an orientation for new employees. Typically this orientation process takes place over a one-to-two day period. The personnel department, staff development, and/or nursing education often run the orientation process. Material covered includes an orientation to the hospital, its vision and mission, and any current initiatives. Also included are information relative to support services available to new employees and mandated training in handling of hazardous materials, infection control, fire safety, sexual harassment, and the use and abuse of alcohol and drugs. Other mandated training is generally conducted at orientation and at other times. You will likely receive an employee handbook and directions to review certain hospital policies. You certainly will be alerted to policies such as professional dress codes and patient confidentiality.

If there is a pastoral care department, you may have colleagues who will provide the departmental orientation. This orientation should provide job specifics including the department's vision, mission, scope of services, and specific initiatives. At this time you should also receive and/or negotiate your specific assignments. You will be informed of your work schedule and/or you will need to devise one that covers the pastoral care needs of the facility. If you are "on call" you will be so notified. Some pastoral care departments have an emergency availability plan instead of a formal "on call." If you are the only person making up pastoral services you may or may not find departmental policies and information available and in place. Should you find yourself without such material, it is a good idea to seek help from colleagues who usually are willing to share. For a sample departmental orientation checklist see Appendix K.

Quality Care Standards and Policies

It is essential to know what standards of pastoral/spiritual care are in the field as a whole as well as what are expected in any given situation. These standards of practice provide a knowledge base that keeps ministry moving in a helpful direction. It is possible for chaplains to have had academic and clinical experiences that do not include learning comprehensive standards for hospital ministry or ways to put these standards into practice. Should you find yourself in need of these resources, whether you are new to hospital ministry or have been in the field for many years, you will find help from chaplains' associations, hospital accreditation services, literature in the field, and professional clinical associations. In Appendix D you will find a sample policy statement of the department of pastoral services in an acute psychiatric facility.

Management of Information

Information is an essential commodity in hospital settings. Chaplains need to know the following:

- Who is in the hospital (admissions, transfers and discharges, census, religious preferences, unit, room, date of admission, length of stay)
- The diagnosis and treatment plan for the patient (access to records and treatment teams)
- Restrictions and expectations
- Contagious or infection control issues
- Attitudes and behaviors that may be of concern
- Special and/or closely monitored treatment plans and/or interventions
- Significant changes in health—particularly life threatening changes
- Preferences by the patient as to the provision or nonprovision of services
- Discharge plans that may indicate the need for further services or referral of services (outpatient clinics, nursing homes, group homes, rehabilitation services, transfers and treatment at other hospitals, home health care)
- Limitations regarding the receipt of the sacrament or ordinance of Holy Communion

Nonverbal Communication

In relationships, most communication is nonverbal. The same is true in hospital ministry, no matter how hard the organization tries to be explicit about its communications. Being able to identify and interpret cues is a knowledge-based skill crucial to any people-based activity. Therefore, it is just as important to pay attention to what is not said as it is to what is said. Often, nonverbal cues are observed through behavior and body language, and by the use of verbal techniques such as questioning, restating, clarifying, and wondering about an observed cue. This observation, understanding, and interpreting, of nonverbal behavior and communication is applicable for ministry with patients, families, visitors, volunteers, colleagues, and staff alike.

Chaplains vary in their ability to pay attention to and utilize nonverbal communication. One student in a second unit of clinical training caught on right away as demonstrated by the choice of the following learning goal, "During this unit I have sought to be aware of verbal cues, body language, and defensive mechanisms during patient visits and staff interactions. I listen not only to the words, but to the meaning behind the words."

Other chaplains and individuals involved in hospital ministry do not pay such close attention. This inattention to nonverbal cues inevitably leads to problems in their ministries. Examples of problems created by inattention to nonverbal clues are:

- Entering a room when the door is closed or a curtain is drawn without knocking or checking with nursing
- Persisting on talking, visiting, and reading scripture when a person turns his or her head aside, looks angry, closes eyes, is sleeping, has difficulty breathing, or gives any indication of having difficulty
- Following a person who has walked or moved away after an introduction
- Not assessing pacing, gesturing, or other signs of behavioral frustration and possible escalation of potentially harmful behavior and strong feelings

These examples constitute misreading or not paying attention to cues. Sometimes this difficulty is an indication of a novice and is easily remedied with skill training. Many hospitals offer this kind of training for other disciplines, and there are ample books and resources designed for self-learning endeavors.

At other times misreading cues can be an indication of conflicting emotional issues that may be occurring within the chaplain. Consistent inattention in situations that involve emotional issues may be an indication of a chaplain being overwhelmed, having strong countertransference responses, being burned-out emotionally, or in need of a consult, or indicate a need for therapy to help resolve feelings and personality issues that may be interfering with effective ministry.

Emotional and personality issues are often identified by risk-taking behaviors including minimization, over-valuation of self and skills, under or over valuation of others, and crossing or being tempted to cross professional boundaries.

Pastoral Care Basics

Pastoral care and counseling is a knowledge or skill-based endeavor. At times, persons in and outside hospital ministry tend to ignore or minimize the body of knowledge available in the field. However, the need for trained professionals is essential to the provision of quality spiritual care services to those in need.

Spiritual Needs

The surveyed students discussed earlier, who were new to hospital ministry, focused on several spiritual needs that they were able to identify in their first unit of clinical training. They realized that they had spiritual and faith experiences they brought with them to the training program and that these experiences could be a rich resource for them later in their careers. They were also learning about being with patients in times of vulnerability. They learned about differing spiritual care needs and faith traditions. In all cases, these basic spiritual needs would become the foundations of a professional identity for them as parish clergy, chaplains, and pastoral counselors.

Faith Experiences

The movement from having a faith experience and using that experience in one's hospital ministry is a journey that can take years. Certainly, experienced chaplains find they continually learn and grow through action and reflection on their ministry. Persons come to ministry with a faith experience that usually becomes a "call" to ministry. In some cases this call is to hospital ministry. The ability to professionally reflect on experiences and find spiritual meaning that contributes to one's faith and beliefs is a skill that can be learned. Common methods for learning about faith experiences are meditation and prayer, journaling, spiritual direction programs, supervised and advanced clinical training, continuing education and consultation.

Faith Connections

Traditionally, hospital chaplains have been expected to be in good standing with a specific faith tradition. Occasionally one finds situations where an individual has some kind of spiritual care training component and engages in hospital ministry without the support or endorsement of their faith tradition. Faith connections are important for helping set standards of ministry, for support and consultation, and for accountability.

Ministry of Presence

When students begin their clinical training they are encouraged to develop an introductory skill known throughout the clinical pastoral discipline as "presence." Therefore, it is not a surprise that the students who brainstormed on the needs of persons new to hospital ministry needed to learn how to show up, be present, and not try to solve problems. This helps a person new to chaplaincy for they often aren't equipped to provide additional sophisticated interventions.

The meaning of "presence" varies from individual to individual, and is perhaps rightly termed as the "art" and "spirit" of pastoral ministry. Pastoral presence usually refers to the making of relational connections that include personal and transpersonal dimensions. To be present is to be open to person and larger context. It is both an active and receptive stance wherein spirit can move and bring meaning and purpose to life. Pastoral presence and sound pastoral practices, when used skillfully together, constitute to two essentials of healing hospital ministry.

"Being 'present' has taken on a broader meaning," states an insightful student, "it means being tuned-in to receive and do God's will for me. Allowing myself to trust the way I am being guided and to reap the benefits of whatever I find is the new dimension that allows me to give to others, not from myself but from God, using me as a conduit. All I have to do is get out of the way and pay attention."

Theological Differences and Differing Faith Traditions

Usually, clinical training opportunities give students exposure to differing faiths and traditions. For example, I remember an advanced unit of clinical pastoral education that I took in a Catholic hospital setting. Most of the patients were Catholic and I was the only non-Catholic student in the peer group. Plus, I was an ordained clergy-woman to boot. I learned a lot about the Catholic faith in that unit. Much of that experience in a predominately Catholic setting still helps me today in my current setting where 50 percent of the patients and staff are Catholic.

It is crucial to acquaint yourself with as many faith traditions and spiritual beliefs and experiences as possible. If you did not get a wide exposure in your clinical training or from your upbringing, you will need to be proactive in learning all that you can. Find out as quickly as possible which faith groups are identified by patients upon admission. If the hospital does not ask for this information upon admission, you will want to suggest that this information be requested. Most hospital departments now have census information about religious preferences. This information is usually available to hospital chaplains and sometimes to parish clergy.

Once you determine the predominant faith groups in your hospital setting you will want to begin learning about religious and spiritual care practices that can be used in times of illness. You will also want to know about any expectations that a specific faith group places on its members. A review of current literature would be helpful as would contact with clergy and faith groups in your area.

Devotional Aids

Devotional aids are those items or objects used to help an individual, family, or group focus on beliefs and connections that provide hope and meaning during times of health care need. These aids differ according to beliefs and faith traditions. It is usually best to ask people what aids, if any, are helpful to them. Chaplains usually build up a knowledge and inventory of these aids. Frequently used items are Holy Scriptures from varying traditions, crosses, relics, statues, pictures, prayer rugs, and literature. Music is also a frequent devotional aid.

Spiritual Practices

The most universally helpful spiritual practice across religions and faith traditions is prayer. This is closely followed by some form of meditation or focused reflection. In addition, practices asked for sometimes involve the availability of communion and the anointing of the sick. Worship services or prayerful chapel spaces contribute to providing a space and a context for spiritual practices.

One student from a free church tradition reflected on the spiritual aspect of prayer: "I am amazed at how many individuals in hospital care keep prayer as a priority. They speak tenderly about their prayer lives and don't necessarily need me to pray with them. After all, God hasn't suddenly arrived with me, but has been here all along. So, my presence gives permission for people to speak out loud about their faith and prayer lives. They share with me the most intimate details about their beliefs. This is very special."

Much of hospital ministry involves helping people stay connected to their spiritual beliefs and practices. In cases where this connection is missing, unhelpful, or inaccessible, the chaplain's role is to facilitate the growth, development, and restoration of spiritual health and practice where possible and desired.

Code of Ethics

Many churches and all clinical pastoral organizations have developed a professional code of ethics for clergy and chaplains. These ethical standards provide guidelines that are intended to ensure that quality services are provided and that persons are neither abused nor neglected in any way. These standards also provide reminders of boundaries and parameters of their work and calling. In addition, the hospital itself has its own standards that apply to all its employees and other persons working within the hospital. While these standards constitute knowledge-based information, they are listed under spiritual needs because chaplains also consider these ethical codes to be morally right and good ways of behaving that usually complement their beliefs and values.

Ethics

In addition to a personal and professional code of ethics applied to individuals, ethical matters are deliberated on involving the specifics of health care for persons in treatment. Chaplains are usually involved as a member of hospital ethics committees and invariably need additional training in health care and medical ethics.

IDENTIFYING PROFESSIONAL MINISTRY NEEDS

It is not possible to describe all of the professional needs a person is likely to encounter in the practice of hospital ministry. To some degree, each setting and individual must shape his or her own ministry style and focus. To this end, an empty chart is included which is intended to be used to reflect on the professional needs of the reader (see Appendix M). After reading this chapter you may want to take the time to copy this chart and fill in your professional needs as you experience them now. As you continue to read this book you may wish to add and make changes to your needs sheet. Completing the sheet will provide you with a working description of your professional needs. Later, you may want to share this information with others in your department. You may invite them to do their own needs profile. You may also wish to construct a profile for your department. By all means share the results with consultants and persons who provide professional support.

Chapter 6
Developing Caring Contexts for Health and Healing

A POEM

"O, My Lord God, I have heartily offended thee . . ."
  His mind will not stop its careening path
  through guilt, fear and apprehension.

"It is too much . . ."
  Over and over again he wanders off
  into the world of repetition which is
  his even though it is unknown to him.

"I'll say it just once between five and seven . . ."
  His voice is loud, conviction firm, as he
  towers over me, his pastor, still hearing
  priests of years gone by.

"But then, I'll slip and do it again . . ."
  "Just once," I say, "and let that be it
  for the day," repeating it twice just
  to be sure. Step on a crack and break
  my mother's back. Sticks and stones
  will break my bones but names will
  never hurt me.

"O, My Lord God, I have heartily offended thee."

CARING CONTEXTS FOR SPIRITUAL HEALING

Certain people, processes, places, and relationships are containers or contexts, and catalysts to care and healing. In order to act as such, the person in need of care must first be able to access these differing contexts within the hospital in ways that promote health and healing. In order for health and healing to occur, life-giving energy must be experienced by the individual in these contexts. From a hospital ministry perspective, this healing, caring, life-giving energy, will heal the spirit of the individual because it promotes physical, mental, emotional and/or sociological healing connections. A model for this approach is presented in Figure 6.1.

THE SELF AS PATIENT AND HEALER

Each of us lives according to the meaning, purpose, or direction we have accumulated in our lives. This spiritual part of ourselves is the sum of our spiritual past. We make meaning of this past and use it to make spiritual choices in the present. Part of this spiritual past is made up of the hopes, wishes, and dreams that are yet to be fulfilled. It is

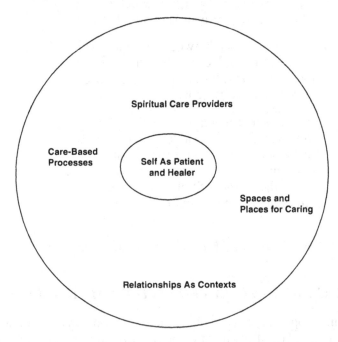

FIGURE 6.1. The Caring Context for Health and Healing Within the Hospital Ministry Setting

these hopes, wishes, and dreams that energize and move us into our future. Our spiritual memories (lived experiences), combined with spiritual sparks (wishes, dreams, and hopes), provide us with a central core of meaning that we rely upon fairly unconsciously from day to day.

Personal Core of Meaning Context

When faced with challenging or new situations such as illness, dysfunction, and hospitalization, we draw from our internal core of meaning in an effort to make sense out of what is happening. When that core is positive, spirit filled, and hopeful, there is a greater ability to make sense of what is happening to us. A person with a constructive and spirit-filled core of meaning has resources when faced with such a need.

Sometimes a person's experiences and memories are fragmented. Their spirits are broken or undeveloped. Their life wishes and dreams are filled with despair. Their hopes are dashed again and again. These persons may find that their core of meaning (their inner spirit) has become so dampened, hidden, or battered, that turning to it leaves them unfulfilled, confused, and depleted. For these individuals, a health crisis such as hospitalization can be quite overwhelming.

In some cases, people find themselves unable to understand and develop as they would like to be able to do. They experience spiritual frustration and may become cynical. They may hide their values and wishes for the duration of their lives; they may focus on the needs of others by helping them fulfill their needs and dreams at the expense of their own. At times they may live vicariously. For these persons, hospitalization and illness are obstacles they have learned to manage, manipulate themselves around without fully recovering from the illness event or handling it well.

Others are seekers and wanderers who never quite settle into a specific life direction. These persons never quite find meaning to lean on for an extended period of time. They are not so much spirit filled or spirit drained, but rather, they have difficulty accessing spirit and meaning in a predictable and reliable way. Hospitalization and illness, for individuals, becomes an interlude on a wandering journey through life. Sometimes these individuals are spiritually lost and don't have the advantage of knowing it. This makes it difficult for true growth and development to happen. Health care, like spiritual care, happens for these people, but in a passive and frequently unplanned way.

Still, most find themselves moving through life with an ability to make some sense of it. Helping patients access, assess, and develop their core of meaning (spirit) is a beginning step to recovery and is at the heart of hospital ministry. Helping patients apply that spirit (core of meaning) to health and illness is crucial to health and healing.

Person in Need of Care and Healing—A Holistic Context

For many years the medical field, and our culture, has considered the primary role of the patient to be the recipient of care. Little attention was paid to the patient's role as a healer. The healer function was reserved for professionals who were trained to perform certain health care functions for, on behalf of, or with the patient. Over time, medical and physical aspects of health care began to take priority over other aspects of health care.

In recent years, we have come to realize that health care is not so easily compartmentalized nor is the healer's role limited to professionals. Abigail Evans, in her recent book, *Redeeming Marketplace Medicine* (1999), is one of the more recent writers who advocates clearly for this concept of "patient as healer" by stating,

> the patient is the central but not the primary healer. The patient is central because she initiates the relationship and enlists other healers. However, once involved in a relationship with professional healers, the patient does not serve as the primary healer. She relies on the expertise and knowledge of the professional. Hence the role of the patient as healer is fluid, but the patient should be actively involved as long as possible. (p. 131)

Evans also advocates for holistic health care. She believes that health "is personal wholeness and healing refers to any activity that moves us toward wholeness, then anyone who contributes to our journey toward health is a healer" (p. 119). These shifts toward holistic and inclusive thinking are not easily made in a system that has pretty much been founded on a hierarchical and territorial model. Even in hospital settings where there is increased awareness of holistic and person-centered healing and healer functions, one finds it very difficult to embrace this way of thinking.

At New Hampshire Hospital, we have also been using a holistic model of personhood and of spiritual needs and resources. The model we have drawn upon in the pastoral services department comes from the work of Beck, Rawlins, and Williams (1988). We teach this model to new employees, students, and patients in some of our therapeutic groups. This model states that persons are made up of five dimensions with needs and resources in each. The five dimensions are:

1. Physical needs
2. Intellectual/mental needs
3. Emotional needs
4. Social needs
5. Spiritual needs

Although hospital ministry addresses all five dimensions of personhood, it specializes in the area of spiritual care. This specialization was recently emphasized by the Pastoral Care Week Committee (FY 2000). According to this committee,

> pastoral care identifies the needs, hopes and resources of each person, collaborates with that person and his or her support system to use spiritual resources for healing and well-being.

According to the Beck model (Beck, Rawlins, and Williams, 1988), every person has spiritual needs, stressors, and resources. These needs, stressors, and resources are found in five spiritual areas. These spiritual areas are identified as need for:

1. A philosophy of life
2. Awareness of the numinous or hope
3. A relationship to God or a higher power
4. Relationship to nature and people
5. Spiritual fulfillment

Spiritual Needs

A Philosophy of Life

An individual's philosophy of life is made up of beliefs, values, morals, and ethics. Often these beliefs are expressed in clichés such as "You get what you deserve," or "What goes around comes around."

Often a philosophy of life is found in "should" and "ought" statements such as "You should do as you are told," or "You ought not to have done that." A person's philosophy of life can also be summed up in repeated phrases and words of wisdom such as, "I find that never works," or "I feel that it is important to tell the doctor everything."

Awareness of the Numinous or Hope

Experiences of emotions, such as awe, or reverence, are also spiritual experiences. An ability to challenge oneself to go beyond one's ordinary everyday limits can be due to a spiritual capacity for hope and transcendence. The rise to consciousness and increased awareness of an unusual experience, and moments of enlightenment that cannot be explained by human reasoning, can be said to be spiritual experiences.

A Relationship to God or a Higher Power

People have a spiritual need to find meaning, and to express ideas and thoughts relating to a supreme being, universal power, or force. The presence of God, the integration of the universe, and the meaning of life, are often evoked through participation in familiar religious rituals and ceremonies. This presence can be cultivated internally and in connection with nature as well as with other people.

Relationship to Nature and People

Our relationships with people may lift our spirits, help us feel connected, and encourage us to develop genuine love and grow in wisdom and compassion. Our relationship with nature may teach us humility, respect, and courtesy. Positive experiences in both areas enlarge our spirit and provide for us a sense of place in this world and universe.

Spiritual Fulfillment

Spiritual fulfillment is experienced when one is able to transcend limitations and to realize one's potential, and also by looking to the horizon and having a sense of vision. Spiritual fulfillment may also happen as one experiences personal power, values, what happens in life, or is transformed and strengthened by life's experiences.

Assessment of Spiritual Needs

While we can use accumulated wisdom gained from professional and personal experience to understand spiritual needs, stressors and resources, it is always wise to ask patients what they think and feel. Often our hypotheses are confirmed and often we are surprised by the responses given. Sometimes we are in the ballpark, so to speak, and sometimes we are way off base in our understanding and interpretation of the patient's experiences and understandings.

Patients Speak Up

In the winter of 2000, patients referred to an admissions group called "Conversations with the Chaplains," and a longer term care group called, "Spirituality and Recovery," were asked to identify what they considered barriers to their spiritual care and recovery. Once identified, the barriers were divided simply into categories of external and internal barriers. External barriers were further divided into problems relating to spiritual care practices and people and relationship issues. Tables 2.1 and 2.2 (see Chapter 2) show the results of this brainstorming activity.

We found that these barriers to spiritual care and recovery were perceived similarly from unit to unit in the hospital. This confirmed the validity of approaching the task of hospital ministry through the identification of common spiritual care needs, stressors, and resources likely to be found in the hospital experience. The patients involved in this experience found it easier to identify barriers and more difficult to identify resources. Difficulties patients may experience in accessing resources, and limiting or managing stressors, becomes a crucial problem for patients, chaplains, and support systems.

A Simple Assessment of Spiritual Needs

Today there are numerous assessments of spiritual care needs. However, these assessments are often home grown. Some are anecdotal and arise from the extensive experiences of chaplains in the field. My current preference is to use an assessment based on the material from Beck, Rawlins, and Williams (1988). This work has been adapted and used by the department of pastoral services at New

Hampshire Hospital for a number of years. A copy of the adapted format is found in Appendix L.

This assessment is normally done in group discussion. To that end, the chaplain needs to remember the five areas of spiritual needs and resources which are, once again a philosophy of life, awareness of the numinous or hope, a relationship to God or a higher power, relationship to nature and people, and spiritual fulfillment. One must also be cognizant of the five dimensions of a whole person, which are physical needs, intellectual/mental needs, emotional needs, social needs, and spiritual needs. It is crucial to be somewhat relaxed when talking about these dimensions and everyone's spiritual needs and resources. Be quite clear that the term "spiritual" is used in its broadest sense. Also, be careful not to be negative about religion or religious practices. This negativity may cause stress and bias the assessment.

The assessment may be given in narrative format and broken up into smaller pieces. If possible, start with an area you feel the patient might experience as more positive rather than beginning where there is likely to be distress. For example, if you know the patient feels close to God, you may wish to start with a question about his or her belief in God. If you believe the person has been quite angry with his or her spouse or children and fussing with the staff, you may wish to ask about relationships later.

However, if time is severely limited, you may want to perform an internal assessment of your own after listening to the patient. You could follow this with statements such as, "Many people feel supported and spiritually uplifted by being out in the fresh air. How are you managing being confined for such a long time?" You would use this approach in a gentle manner while realizing that even a gentle approach is apt to be seen as confrontational by the patient. A person who has difficulty getting outside, for example, may experience spiritual stressors in many other spiritual needs areas. All assessments are intended to be supportive, even if they serve the purpose of helping individuals face difficult issues. The primary purpose of a spiritual care assessment is to help the patient identify his or her spiritual resources. Remember, the patient is his or her own best team member on many occasions. Spiritual resources can be of great help during hospitalization.

Second, a spiritual care assessment can help a patient identify areas that may be interfering with health and healing, both now and in the future. Some of these stressors can be addressed while the person is in the hospital. At other times the chaplain can help by providing temporary or lasting relief by just listening and working with the patient. Other stressors may need to be set aside as much as possible, and/or perhaps they will need to be neutralized by teaching the patient temporary coping techniques.

THE SPIRITUAL CARE PROVIDER

Developing a Professional Pastoral Care Context

When in-care students are installed in the Merrimack Association of the United Church of Christ in the New Hampshire Conference, each is called to a specific church to be "pastor and teacher." These students have been trained to understand the pastoral caregiving function as a part of ministry. They, along with most other ministers, rabbis, and priests, think of pastoral caregiving as focusing on shut-ins, those who are sick and hospitalized, and families in distress. Sometimes they think of individuals who are imprisoned, refugees, or the homeless who are also in need of pastoral/spiritual care.

Care-Based Interpretation of the Living Human Document

Jeanne Stevenson Moessner, in *Through the Eyes of Women: Insights for Pastoral Care* (1996), describes the typical caregiving view. She says, "Pastoral caregivers have traditionally viewed the individual as a 'living human document' " (p. 7). In fact, we made great progress when we learned to think this way. It caused us to listen to people and really strive to hear their stories and understand where they were coming from and wanting to go. We encouraged individuals to tell us about themselves and what was important to them. We agreed with Anton Boisen, who pointed out to clergy and students the importance of human experience and coined the phrase, "Living Human Document." Mr. Boisen's first use of the term was as early as 1930 (Gerkin, 1984, pp. 37-54).

The Use of Self

The clinical educational task of the chaplain-in-training (when focused on the Living Human Document) in the early years became one of understanding and interpreting the internal experience of "the pastoral self" and the internal experiences of the "patient-other." Once understood and interpreted, the pastoral self and the patient self were assumed to be stronger and better able to manage whatever happens. Self-reflection became a valued tool for chaplains and ministers-in-training. A self that reflected upon itself was considered more integrated and possibly more highly developed. Most ministry was accomplished on a one-to-one basis during those early years, and looked very much like a theological version of Freudian or Jungian therapy, and later on, of object relations work. (Gerkin, 1984). Feelings and perceptions were buried treasure and prized as part of recovery.

Care-Based Context of the Living Human Web

In 1996 we find persons such as Jeanne Stevenson Moessner lifting up the idea of a broader context for pastoral care. She writes:

> Bonnie Miller-McLemore carefully illustrates the pastoral theological shift from a focus on care as counseling the individual as "living human document" to care as part and parcel of a broad social, religious, cultural, and economic context. . . . the metaphor of 'living human web' better represents an understanding of the person-in-relationship. This relatedness includes not only other persons but connectedness with society, family systems, public policy, institutions, and ideologies. (Moessner, 1996, p. 7)

The Living Human Web metaphor for pastoral care has grown out of our understandings of systems and the internal relational processes of women such as is found in self-in-relation theory. Rather than reducing our knowledge of self and of personhood, one prizes any efforts to understand broader connections and interrelations. The Living Human Web is just like a pebble thrown into a pond—it swirls outward. In the context of the Living Human Web, it is just as important to understand interpersonal, cultural, social, and political systems, as it is to understand internal experiences, thoughts, and feelings. The Living Human Web concept of pastoral care is born in the twenty-first century's living global village.

Use of Context

In contextual care theory the pastoral care provider and the patient are part of the same context. When the services provided are in a hospital system, the services needed are no longer confined to the individual person or the individual household. For example, Social Services once focused on family issues and maybe issues of work, household relationships, and support. In many hospitals today there is no such thing as a Department of Social Services. Instead it is called Community Integration. This is what is meant by contextual thinking. If we were honest, we would go even further and consider the health-giving effects of global integration.

Part of the pastoral care provider's job, as part of the human web, is to help other voices be heard. Those who are weaker, less valued, and less powerful are in particular need of being heard. Also in need of being heard are those who think and act differently. The context of pastoral care is no longer primarily "the patient," but rather, the connective and disconnected life in which the patient is currently living.

Readiness to Assist in Care and Healing

Readiness is not a constant state. It is a process. For a provider to be in a state of readiness to assist in care and healing, he or she must have moved through some predictable phases and successfully negotiated key processes along the way. Also, he or she must periodically assess and reassess readiness throughout his or her lifespan as a spiritual care provider. Some predictable processes and stages are described in Table 6.1. These phases are best completed at least one time through before practicing chaplaincy on one's own. However, as with all stage theory, the professional person may have to revisit certain key processes throughout their professional lifespan.

A Student's Experience

Elizabeth came to the hospital for an internship in counseling as part of a psychology practicum. She needed to have 600 clinical hours, including approved supervision. She was interested in holistic

TABLE 6.1. Phases of Readiness

Phases	Progression of Key Process			
Contemplation	Awareness	Experience	Predisposition	Call
Preparation	Training-academic	Training-clinical	Internal correspondence with desire	Connecting and resources
Action	Awareness of needs of others	Provision of skilled services	Internal correspondence with external action	Representation or connection with Divine Other or sacred
Reflection	Insight	Learning	Motivation	Commitment and connectedness

counseling and especially interested in incorporating spiritual care into her counseling. Elizabeth had spent numerous years in the health care system but had had no formal experiences in counseling. At the conclusion of sixty hours of internship, and an especially challenging afternoon consisting of first sessions with three severely traumatized patients, she left supervision declaring with somewhat painful humor, "I say to myself, 'How did I ever get into this!' "

A Care Readiness Questionnaire

In Appendix M, one will find a brief Care Readiness Questionnaire. It would be helpful to complete this questionnaire at one's leisure. For those persons new to hospital ministry, the questionnaire and Table 6.1 will help in the identification of key processes completed.

The effect of using both the chart and the questionnaire will probably have a normalizing effect on those already engaged in hospital ministry. Experienced chaplains and spiritual care providers may want to see these instruments as leading toward a reflective review process. This review can be energizing, empowering, and informative.

CARE-BASED PROCESSES

Service Opportunities As Caring Contexts

A Priest's Experience in Hospital Ministry

Father came to work at the hospital after a number of years in parish ministry. He wanted to be placed in the hospital and looked forward to the ministry possibilities. He got along well with patients, staff, and colleagues. He made rounds and paid attention to those who sought him out, and to those who were referred. Admittedly, he hated paperwork and suffered through meetings. Goodness knows, he couldn't stand the hospital's need to know where he was every minute of the day. Mostly he was a good sport and took a positive view of life and work. He stayed a few years and then went elsewhere. For years afterward, he held affectionate memories of a number of patients and many staff. The frustrating aspects of working in hospital ministry gave way to the ups and downs of the parish. A number of patients and staff in the hospital remembered him affectionately and wished him well. All in all it was a good ministry.

Processes in Readiness to Assist in Care and Healing

Father was ready for hospital ministry. It showed in his choice, in his preparation, and in his actions while in ministry. Although he thoroughly disliked meetings and what he considered to be red tape—setting long-term goals, and anything that took him away from "the people"—he learned to make use of some processes quite effectively. He especially liked the way some processes, such as admissions brochures, rounds, and responding to direct requests and referrals provided a reliable context for care and healing.

Since Father's days of hospital ministry, these processes have become even more sophisticated. Experience dictates that it is crucial to have processes in place for hospital ministry to be efficient and effective. When such processes are in place, they can be immensely helpful context-containers for health, healing, and spiritual care opportunities.

Admission Processes

When a patient is admitted to a hospital it is helpful to have the following incorporated in the admission process:

- A pastoral care brochure (see brochure sample in Appendix I)
- A chaplain request form (see request form sample in Appendix B)
- A census that states, at minimum, the patient's religious preference (see examples of preference choices in Appendix N)

Also crucial are:

- A place on the treatment form or care plan that identifies any faith connection, tradition, religious affiliation, or spiritual beliefs or practices
- A place for notation if a chaplain visit is requested or declined—normally in the progress notes of the patient's record or perhaps in a nursing care plan

Rounds

There are differences in opinion about the use of rounds as an opportunity for pastoral care. The medical model is based on this process of brief daily contact between doctor/nurse and patient. This model is so engrained in all of our thinking that it is a common practice for chaplains to engage in rounds as frequently as possible.

However, it is not always possible for a chaplain to visit each patient. Unlike other professional services who are assigned to a specific ward or unit, the hospital chaplain has a caseload that may or may not be shared with other chaplains. Still, an occasional impromptu visit to a unit is an excellent opportunity for care. In multiple staff situations it may be helpful to have a schedule of rounds. The concept of making rounds, thus becomes a process that contains the idea that pastoral care is available and accessible to all. This makes even the idea of "rounds" a care-based process.

Requests and Referrals

The most effective method for encouraging and managing patient requests is through a specific form that indicates services available (see request form, Appendix B). However, it is crucial to let staff and patients know how to request services from the chaplain and/or the pastoral care department. Preferred methods are:

- Chaplain's request form left at nursing station
- Verbal request to staff who follow up with a call to chaplain
- In-person requests of patients directly to chaplain

Possible barriers:

- Staff decision not to forward request
- Staff forgetting to mention request when chaplain is seen

Referrals are usually requests for services made by staff, family, or significant others. Referrals may also come from other chaplains and health care providers. As a rule, referrals are usually made in the following ways:

- Formal referral for services signed by physician
- Formal referral given orally by any member of the treatment team
- Formal referrals for therapy group services by team
- Consensus driven referral while chaplain is on team

These referrals are given verbally, on pieces of paper, on forms, over the phone, and by e-mail. All referrals require some kind of feedback to the team/referral source when the source is in the hospital setting. In situations where feedback can only be provided with the patient's consent, concerns of confidentiality would dictate responses chosen.

SPACES AND PLACES FOR CARING

Care-Based Spaces That Assist in Care and Healing

More and more we are aware of the impact that milieu has on care and healing. The modulation of light, color, air quality, and space all contribute to health care effectiveness. Much of hospital ministry takes place in the patient's room, in family/visitor rooms, in hallways, and in cafeterias.

Chapels and devotional spaces are especially important as they are set aside with the intention of promoting spiritual healing. These spaces are formally designated for promotion of spiritual care and healing. As such, they are expected to be contexts that are perpetually ready for the assigned task. When they are not, or cannot be immediately made ready, they become barriers rather than carriers of care and meaning.

Chapels

Hospital chapels are prime spaces set aside to promote spiritual care and healing. This dedicated space is symbolic of the essence of spiritual care and resources, hence, the careful use of symbols and other resources sources for meditation and prayer. Additional resources consist of new and timely devotional aids that the chapel visitor may hold or take with them. Prayer cards are helpful—if there is a sense of movement and dedication in the use and producing of these cards. A lively and seasonal changing of the chapel décor promotes the sense of theological story and the spiritual movement of life including a relationship with nature, self, and with divine other. An open-door policy is essential to promote the notion that one is always welcome and that coming and going forth is expected. Chapels must be used for sacramental and worship purposes if they are to be containers of life. Banners and fresh flowers are appreciated. These may flow out into the halls—with life and spirit that connect through those open doors to the rest of the hospital.

A Patient Reflects

Patients, families, visitors, and staff, all bring their thoughts and feelings to the chapel. Often, only the individuals and the divine know these thoughts and feelings. On rare occasion, at least in a psychiatric facility, one can pass by the chapel and be privileged to hear musings. Such was my experience on an afternoon in December.

CHAPEL LISTENING
ON A RAINY, SLEETING AFTERNOON IN DECEMBER

There should be
a Christmas tree
in here,
    maybe in the back
    a crèche.

I don't know all the words,
I have
brain cancer.

I'll be back
to sit
with a friend.

A chapel that invites open-minded thinking and human feelings is crucial to hospital ministry and to health care recovery. This particular patient felt quite at home in this chapel and was able to remember what would be commonly found in church settings at the time of year. Also crucial was the patient's confession of weakness and limitations, and a desire to bring human and divine companionship into the space. The space was clearly user-friendly for this person.

Sometimes what goes on in a chapel does not meet the wishes and needs of certain individuals. However, even in such instances, there can be growth in connection and insight concerning spiritual care practices and preferences. Such was the case for a student intern in a general hospital setting. What follows are this person's written reflections about the hospital chapel as space and service.

A Chaplain Intern's Reflection on Chapel

A lot of times I find chapel annoying. There is often this low-church Protestant thing which if I am honest with myself I find annoying. Of course, I often use the same structure—I can annoy myself—but I guess I'm looking for more structure and richness, and more connection with history.

Chapel Spaces Remembered

Every chaplain has his or her memories of hospital chapels and responses to those devotional spaces. It is a helpful process to reflect on the effect hospital chapels have had on you as a person and as a professional. The following list comes to one chaplain's mind. Ask yourself what your list would include.

- A local small-town general hospital chapel—quiet, tiny, with dead, dried brown flowers as an overwhelmingly large centerpiece.
- A large state hospital for 1,000 elderly persons—chapel services on the wards, no designated space.
- A Roman Catholic general hospital in a moderately large town—with stained glass, stations of the cross, and blond 1950s pews. A central TV system to broadcast services. Overhead announcements of Hail Mary prayers and Holy Communion delivered daily on the wards.
- A state psychiatric facility in a small town—new building with small square space built by architects with no input from chaplains—square ceiling and overhead skylight, with weavings

similar to those found in bank downtown. Added by chaplains were symbols created by Jewish artist (representing Christian and Jewish symbols), a banner pole, a bench from the old chapel, a communion table, paraments, banners, literature, fresh flowers, and an angel carving. The space is kept open for all as devotional space.

- A large general hospital with outstanding reputation—chapel dark and gloomy, poorly identified with dried, dead flowers, with prayer basket and look of no one ever entering place. Door closed.
- Another large general hospital with modest reputation—same as above but with no prayer basket.

Keeping the Chapel Space As a Context for Spiritual Care

Today's chapel spaces must serve many purposes and many traditions. Therefore, it takes concerted foresight and planning to design something that will fit the spiritual care needs of as many patients as possible. Even so, the sacredness of the chapel space can be challenged in unexpected ways.

In many cases, the larger hospital world may try to infringe on the chapel space in ways that threaten its existence. This is often so because today's hospital is often a place where space is at a premium. Many persons and groups vie for that space. Some of its uses are not appropriate.

For example, often the chapel is placed out of the way, which can be problematic. One chapel that was left unlocked after dayshift hours was used for forced and consenting sexual encounters. That chapel door had to be locked during second and third shifts as a result. During those hours, access to the chapel needed to go through security, a necessary but frustrating decision for all.

Every now and then, some hospitals find that staff huddle in the chapel space to work on treatment issues. Sometimes groups will think of the chapel space as a meeting room and request its use. But mostly, with diligence on the chaplaincy's part, persons come and go, kneel at the communion table or the cross, sit and hum, or are found tucked behind the door reading meditational material. This is the life that the hospital chapel is meant to have. This is its healing context and its spirit-filled service!

Quiet Spaces

One of the recent patient surveys conducted in a psychiatric hospital revealed interesting feedback from discharged consumers. Almost 30 percent indicated that they had difficulty finding peace and quiet when they needed it during their hospitalization. For those who work in psychiatric settings, such issues can be challenging on a given unit. However, a recent conversation with a chaplain from a general hospital brought insight to the shared problem of peace and quiet. In these settings there is much activity, comings and goings, tests, transportation, and the general hum of active health care settings. Peace and quiet are apparently essential to some patients' recovery, and are essential components for spiritual care practices such as prayer and meditation. However, peace and quiet are hard to find in hospitals.

Luckily, the chaplain's office is often a quiet space. There are times, in fact, when I have invited staff to feel free come into my office to be alone. At times I sit silently while patients think, feel, and reflect in relative peace. They come to my office for its beauty: the light from the large window and the devotional pictures and symbols of differing faiths and of the sea.

A Quiet Space for Feelings

Quiet places allow thoughts and feelings to flow. This happens frequently when a person feels safe and comfortable. I remember writing a poem about a young twenty-three-year-old who found the space to feel in my office one quiet afternoon.

SILENT TEARS

I lean one hand
on arm
no longer straight
as in my youth

to hear those silent tears
of loveless years
gone bad
beyond all recognition.

A Quiet Space for Talk

Sometimes quiet spaces give a person permission to speak. Giving voice to thoughts and feelings is not always easy. This was especially true for a man in his mid-life years. Just being his own witness to lack of voice was a healing step for this patient. Putting his words into poetry helped me to hear him.

PRIVATE TALK

> I am a private person
> used to keeping things
> to myself
> that's the way I was raised.
> A man is a man.
>
> So I let things build
> and build they did
>
> 'Til I was overwhelmed.
> Now they say things will
> be different. We talk.

A Quiet Space for Being Alone

The hospital itself can be amazingly noisy. However, there are times, such as third shift, weekends, and other unexplained moments, when the hospital can be unbelievably quiet. These quiet times can be an opportunity to reflect on the sounds of the surrounding world. This can be a good thing, for spiritual care involves the capacity to be alone and the capacity to experience the unknown or mystery. I discovered such an epiphany one Christmas day:

A SILENT CHRISTMAS VIGIL

> Sometimes it is so quiet and peaceful
> a scream here,
> a door click,
> the elevator bell,
> a cart, then voices speaking
> sounds—words not identified
> with meaning.
> Tears,
> overhead calling, ah, again a
> friend, the elevator bell.

Makeshift Environments

A chair in the hall, a spot at the end of the unit by a window, a bench strategically placed outside in the afternoon sun—these are spaces that encourage people to sit, to talk, and to meditate. Frequently, it is the task of the chaplain to identify spaces that are conducive to conversation or other spiritual care practices. These makeshift spaces can provide room for the soul to heal.

When patients' rooms are busy, and often filled with two or more people, a curtain can be drawn slightly, or all the way, to give the feeling of space. With permission from other staff, a patient may be moved to a quiet spot. Even a walk or ride outside, physical condition warranting, can provide nature's room and enhance healing. A chaplain must be ready and willing to help each patient find places within the hospital that promote spiritual healing.

Twenty-First-Century Technology: Phones, Computers, and E-Mail

Some spaces, people, relationships, and contexts transcend time and place. We used to think this was so in memory and in our hopeful imaginations, for it is commonly known that we internalize the experiences and memories of people within ourselves. Had the person in the following poem had more money or access to advanced technology I would have probably received this message by e-mail.

A PATIENT'S PHONE CALL

The call came in the early afternoon.
A voice said "Hello,"
and there was silence.

I waited
then said,
"May I ask who this is?"

Don't you remember me?
It's been five years.
I'm in a safe place.

I just had to hear your voice
I'm feeling so alone and
you will always be my Reverend McCall.

It is amazing to realize that caring spiritual contexts will be enhanced through new technologies. But think, do you go through any one day without coming across someone using a cell phone? Do you go through one business day without receiving a fax or e-mail? Does there exist anyone under sixty who does not know about the Internet and the growing use of chat rooms or the relationships blooming there? Is there anyone under sixty who has not heard that some people are able to be connected through the computer to their doctors? Instant access! Within twenty years these contexts will be primary places for caring, health, and healing, if the technology is handled well.

Today I receive requests for services, referrals, and concerns over the e-mail. The time will come when these services will be accessible to hospitalized patients on their units. No longer will they need to rely on word-of-mouth communication and paper-based forms. No longer will they have difficulty getting spiritual are providers of their faith tradition to make visits. They will have access to virtual reality visits and interactions on their computers or TVs.

RELATIONSHIPS AS CONTEXTS

In the case of the ex-patient whose call served the purpose of reassurance and reconnection, one might say that he or she was seeking a relational checkup. For some time, professionals in the counseling field have been aware of the dynamic known as internalization of the therapist. In successful insight oriented therapy, the patient is said to take unto self many aspects of the therapist and of the therapeutic relationship. This internalized relationship is said to have residual positive effects over time. Such was the case of this young person who internalized this relationship to such a degree that it could be counted on some five years later.

Spiritually Transforming Relationships

Not all relationships are contexts for spiritual transformation, but each contact has an opportunity for embodying profound change. Notable relational opportunities for profound spiritual transformation and healing in hospital ministry are:

- The self relates to authentic other
- The self relates to caring family/community
- The self relates to caring and skilled professionals
- The self relates to pastoral caregiver
- The self relates to Holy/divine other

Example: A Relationship at Work

Authentic caring and skill-based relationships are at the heart of healing. Therefore, understanding the various resources available in relationships is crucial to hospital ministry. In the following poem, the patient struggles with the chaplain as representative of parental and divine functions, and comes to a sense of resolution, for the moment, and is temporarily at peace.

DOING WHAT IS ASKED

He enters weakly
asking to sit.
I, an arm leaning,
respond and wait.

Leaning back in chair
he asks if perchance he is
possessed
or so someone has said.

Considering carefully,
his words and sound intention
I tell him, "no."
It doesn't cost me much.

Leaning forward,
he now proclaims, in anguish
deep and moving,
"I try to do what you tell me to do."

At a loss, I search the past
and cannot remember telling him
to do or not to do anything
and so I say, "Do You?"

He seems to rest, leaning back
he thinks real hard
and comes to light,
"I know,
I'll try to do better."

The Self Relates to Authentic Other

Relationships that promote healing are of prime interest to health care providers. Not all relationships are equal, however. Authentic relationships are thought to be contexts for potential healing due to their grounding in common humanity. These healing relationships are best described as consisting of moments where the core spirit of self somehow touches the core spirit of another. Such contexts are filled with energy and the possibility for being oneself more fully. When it is difficult to help a patient find such a relationship, other more scary feelings develop and create less optimum conditions for healing.

Example

Charlene is an attractive middle-aged woman who has difficulty managing her anxieties, and every so often needs hospitalization to help stabilize her medical condition. She normally takes good care of herself and maintains a job that she enjoys. This morning she was doing well and expecting to be discharged. She wanted to talk to a chaplain and was delighted to see one. She spoke of her discharge and of her need to be more independent and more assertive. One of her greatest challenges, from her perspective, was how to relate to her adult child who kept treating her like a child. One of her dearest wishes was to have this adult child listen to her, and empathize with her about the medical challenges she faced. Instead, whenever she shared her anxiety, the adult child would give her impatient fix it answers.

The Self Relates to Caring Family/Community

It is possible to have close and caring relationships within one's nuclear family and have other troubled and nonsupportive relationships elsewhere. These extended relationships can function as health stressors and health resources. Relationships with family and within one's community are crucial to feeling at home in the world. The positive and nurturing context of feeling at home occurs when one is allowed to be oneself, to contribute, to learn, and to grow. Sometimes, being oneself means being ill and needing help to recover.

Transformative relationships that promote healing within family and community are essential. Therefore, a chaplain's task includes helping families learn, grow, and change in their beliefs and in ways their beliefs are practiced in family and community.

The Self Relates to Caring and Skilled Professionals

The hospital community functions best when it is both skilled and professional in its approach to patient care. One of the great mysteries in health care is the essential relationship correlation between skill and care. Therefore, helping professional relationships are those that relate to the individual and to the illness simultaneously.

Example

Charles was hospitalized for bypass surgery. The plan was that he would be in the hospital for several days and go home for the rest of his recovery. Nurses came frequently to check on Charles while he was hospitalized. He could tell that they were merely doing their jobs, and all was proceeding like clockwork. Mostly he remained quiet, did what he was told, and tried to learn what he would need to do when he got home. But his wife was worried and asked question after question of staff. After a couple of days, it was clear that the staff were getting a bit worn down. By the third day, different nurses started coming to check on Charles and do what needed to be done. Each time, each nurse would smile and patiently answer Charles' wife's questions that had already been asked numerous times. Each nurse would reassure Charles' wife. As Charles discovered that the nurses had found a way to relate to his anxious wife, and were doing so caringly and constructively, he became visibly more relaxed and more conversational himself. He went home on time and in a hopeful mood.

The Self Relates to Pastoral Caregiver

Patients expect chaplains to be friendly and respectful. They expect chaplains to listen and to be empathic. They expect chaplains to know something about religion and spiritual care. The healing bonus in this relationship happens when the chaplain, within the realm of professional boundaries, can be both human and humane. This is such a positive and refreshing experience for patients that they often feel free to be more open and honest in the relationship.

The Self Relates to Holy/Divine Other

In the Christian tradition, God resolves the challenge of humanity by changing the relationship to a fully living context where self lives with divine other in healing and therefore saving ways. This, of course, is the message of incarnational care. The work of hospital ministry is to do likewise by building relationship bridges that promote positive contact and positive contexts for healing.

In summary, from a spiritual care and healing perspective, people, processes, and relationships are all resources for promoting healing and recovery from illness. The clinically trained chaplain is typically a trained professional who sees the person and the world holistically, and by doing so, breaks down territorial assumptions that may create barriers to health and healing. This frees up more resources for healing and promotes individualized services. True efforts to develop caring contexts for healing are not necessarily neat, orderly, or predictable processes. Perhaps this is why they have such power to motivate and change lives.

Chapter 7

Focusing on Skill Development

My daughter mulches completely differently than I . . . She, in the service of some five-year-old muse, picks up small hands of grass clippings and, like a fairy princess dusting with stardust, places a few of the clippings gently on the head of a Montauk daisy. She then walks the five hundred feet back to the clipping pile, picks up another handful of grass clippings and, muttering magical incantations, dusts a day lily or pea pod. She says she is going to start on the raspberries tomorrow, a project that should take her several hundred years. (Schaper, 1995, pp. 5-6)

I asked a colleague who has been a chaplain for twenty-two years, "What are the basic skills unique to hospital ministry?" He sat quietly and thought. He munched on his sandwich and glanced out the office window. After several very quiet moments he declared, "It's hard to remember back that far to the beginning. It's hard to think about early skills when you've been using them so long."

THE ART AND SKILL OF HOSPITAL MINISTRY

Hospital ministry, like any other field, is both art and skill. Most skills can be learned with motivation and practice. However, not everyone who is motivated to learn and practice hospital ministry is skilled. In this sense, skill has to do with the sequences of behaviors that make up the specific tasks required to be knowledgeable and proficient in a field. Once one is skilled in a field, one is said to have the ability to do what needs to be done and demonstrates that ability in a manner that can be confirmed by others who are also skilled in the field.

The art of ministry is often gained through exposure and modeling. Reflection on what one sees and experiences can lead to an internalized, and somewhat intuitive sense of the job. Persons who do not catch on quickly, or don't get the knack of how to engage in hospital ministry right away, can be compared to technicians. They do what they are told, or what they think needs to be done until they acquire some nuances that cause them to work more naturally. One can do a job that is technically right (skill based) but not good (artfully executed), and therefore not produce optimum outcomes. Furthermore, all the desire in the world will not be sufficient to produce a skilled chaplain. Such is the paradox of hospital ministry.

Elsewhere in this book we have reviewed much of the philosophy and processes involved in hospital ministry. We have looked at hospitalization from the patient's point of view, the health care field's perspective, and that of the hospital organization, along with the practical needs of chaplains. This chapter will focus on basic pastoral care skills. Every effort is made to make this chapter practical. Therefore, we begin with what can be called commonsense care strategies and move toward more complex care functions, such as brief supportive counseling and crisis ministry.

Each pastoral care skill area will be identified with a statement about the skill and an example of how that skill is applied in a pastoral care moment. The reader will be able to consider how strong he or she is in each identified skill. Those who assess themselves as low—perhaps due to not paying attention—or not being as good as they would like to be—in the identified skill, will be encouraged to review the suggestions provided at the end of each skill area.

USING COMMON SENSE

Being the Stranger

It takes skill to enter into new relationships with people for the purpose of offering professional help. In hospital ministry, we continuously visit strangers. We do this as part of our job. We do this as part of our call and as part of our values and beliefs.

Pastorally, Christian chaplains remember Jesus' words about being a stranger:

For I was hungry and you gave me food, I was thirsty and you gave me drink, I was a stranger and you welcomed me, I was naked and you clothed me, I was sick and you visited me, I was in prison and you came to me. (Matthew 25:35-36)

We visit patients who are strangers to us and we have a theological reason for doing so. We visit in the name of Jesus, if we are Christian. We do this even when we do not name the theological basis of what we are doing and thereby respect differing beliefs.

Chaplains of other faith traditions draw on their traditions for examples and admonitions to visit and care for strangers who become hospitalized. For example, according to *Gates of Prayer,* "These are the obligations without measure, whose reward, too, is without measure . . . to welcome the stranger; to visit the sick . . ." (Stern, 1982 p. 683).

Example

A newly admitted patient was having difficulty handling a series of recent losses. The nurse recognized that treatment and genuine recovery for this patient would need to involve some kind of one-to-one counseling. So she asked the hospital chaplain, a licensed pastoral psychotherapist, to see what could be done. Upon introduction to the patient, the chaplain tried to set up a time to talk. The patient declined to talk at the moment and, when pressed, set a time for forty-five minutes later. The chaplain returned to find that the patient was in tears and had just been speaking with an aid while playing a game. It was then that it occurred to this chaplain just how much of a stranger professionals are in people's lives. So the chaplain, having realized this, used the realization to align with the patient by saying, "It must be difficult to have to talk about yourself to so many strangers." The patient nodded and moved from a resistant stance to one of open sharing.

How to Develop This Skill

- Put yourself in the person's place in order to develop greater empathy.
- Consider your beliefs around the care and visitation with strangers.

- Reflect on feelings you have surrounding such visits and consult openly with a trusted colleague.
- Prepare for visits by thinking the visit through; role playing difficult types of visits; coming up with a typical visit that you would be comfortable doing.
- During the visit, use active imagery or self-talk to create a feeling within yourself of warmth toward the person you are visiting. Adjust your nonverbal behaviors accordingly.

Promoting Hospitality

According to Melanie Rowlison, hospitality involves "a love of strangers, creating an environment where people feel valued and cared for, welcomed, safe, and comfortable—where relationships can develop and persons are at ease, even in unfamiliar surrounding" (Halverson, 1999, p. 71). The ability to create, promote, and embody hospitality is an art that comes naturally to some persons and must be learned by others. One of the tasks of hospital chaplains is to help ease the anxiety and pain one feels when away from home, facing health issues, and in need of a stranger's help in order to recover.

In today's business world, the notion of hospitality is absorbed in what is called customer service. The provision of customer service means that every effort is made to meet or exceed the expectations of customers. Of course, in the business world, the primary reason for providing outstanding customer service is to ensure that customers will not only come back for further services, but will let others know what wonderful services they received. The organization gets the additional benefit of pride of accomplishment.

Hospitality, in the Jewish and Christian sense, is a notion based on the goodness inherent in all of creation. We have a reverence for all that God has made and a sense of the belonging and interconnectedness of all of life. Further, we are to be receptive to those in need. Again, just as in the notion of the stranger, we do so on behalf of God.

Example

The hospital chapel is filling with patients ready for Sunday morning worship service. As people gather, the chaplain welcomes them saying, "It's good to have you all here. This is a chapel of all faiths and we welcome you and all people to this service knowing that there are a variety of traditions and beliefs. Everyone is welcome as we join together in a spirit of worship. Should others come after we start we will want to welcome them too."

How to Develop This Skill

- Imagine yourself as host or hostess in your own home and reflect on the preparations you make when you know someone is coming to your house. Also imagine what you say and how you behave.
- Next, imagine how you like to be treated when you go for a checkup or interact with someone from the medical field.
- Reflect on the chaplains or clergy that you have known and consider what you did and didn't like about their pastoral care approach.
- List ways that you let patients know how you value and care for them.
- What do you do that helps a patient feel safe with you?
- In what ways do you arrange your office so that persons will feel welcomed?
- Visit a hospital that you have never visited. Wander around. Ask if they have a chapel and a chaplain. Notice how people respond and what the environment looks like.

Embodying Respect

Sometimes I hear people say they have been disrespected. In the everyday tongue this means they have been put down. It is actually all too easy in the hospital setting to treat patients in condescending ways. It is not that we mean to do so, but we have the power to intervene in their lives at a time when they are feeling powerless. To respect another is to regard that person as highly as you do yourself. In cases where you don't respect yourself very highly, and suffer from low self-esteem, you may need personal help before you are able to be genuinely respectful of others.

Example

A colleague of mine comes from another country. Recently, he and I were talking about the way we treat patients. We both agreed that sometimes we were not as respectful as we should be. He helped me think about my own pastoral approach when he said, "I call every patient by the title of Mr., Mrs., or Miss. I believe that is a more respectful way to be helpful and professional."

How to Develop This Skill

- Think first of the strengths of the people for whom you are providing care.
- Take a self-help test to inform you about the health of your own self-esteem.
- Practice affirming something about everyone you meet.

Practicing Kindness

In the medical world there is a physician's creed to "do no harm." In Jewish and Christian scriptures, we see that God has shown great kindness to us when we act in less than kind ways toward ourselves and others. Kindness in hospital ministry involves caring and respecting people. It involves thinking of ways to be helpful. Kindness clearly means not harming or doing bad, mean, or hurtful things to others.

Example

A man came by my office one day and asked me to tell him what happens after someone dies. I asked him what he believes happens. He said, "Well, there is a heaven and there is a hell. But tell me the truth, Reverend." I knew that this person felt he had done some pretty unforgivable things. I knew he had prayed for forgiveness for many years. I also knew he had been very sick when he had done those things. We had talked about this through the years. So, this time I decided purposefully to be kind, and responded, "I don't know; you and I won't know for sure until we die. But until then we can live by faith." "What is faith?" he asked. "What we believe," I answered. "I believe we go to heaven," he said and his concerned brow softened as he left. Theology and salvation aside, it seemed a kind thing to ease a bit of his suffering that early morning in September.

How to Develop This Skill

- Practice listening more than talking
- Look for the spirit and not just the theological stance

- Practice seeing yourself as not able to judge
- Imagine yourself as offering warmth and companionable presence
- Give authentic verbal affirmation whenever possible
- Ask the person what would be helpful—this is a kind thing to do

Being Empathic

According to *Webster's* dictionary, empathy is "the capacity for experiencing as one's own the feelings of another" (p. 163). In clinical pastoral education training, the student practices empathy through relating to peers in a structured group setting and through role-playing pastoral care situations. There is no right or wrong way of responding in these situations. However, they require the student to put themselves in different roles and experience as fully as possible the thoughts and feelings they might have under such circumstances. Empathy requires the ability to imagine, connect, and use interior feelings and responses to self and other. It is not an easy skill to acquire, particularly if it is not automatic in the person going into pastoral care or counseling.

Example

The young man was in his bed and quite depressed. He could only seem to think about what had been going wrong for him and how life did not seem all that worthwhile. He felt teary but dared not cry. On that particular day, the equally young chaplain came to the door with a lightness and joy in his step. He was just graduating from seminary and moving on to his first parish. He had the world to live for. The chaplain asked the young man how he was doing. The young man said, "Not well." Then the young man started to list all that had been going wrong. He talked and talked, and as he talked, some of those unwanted tears came to his eyes. The young chaplain listened and found that his heart was feeling heavy too. He thought this young man seemed to have just too much to bear. So he let the young man talk. After twenty minutes the young man said, "Thank you. It was very helpful to get these thoughts off my chest." The young chaplain murmured, "I know you are having a difficult time. I am available to listen or be helpful in any way that I can." After a brief prayer the chaplain left the room.

How to Develop This Skill

- Empathy requires listening, hearing, and providing some kind of feedback in a way that the other person perceives as deep understanding of the thoughts and feelings being expressed. Practice all three components regularly in care visits.
- Empathy is built on the foundation of accurately identifying feelings being expressed, explicit or implied. If you are not sure, ask people what they are feeling and internally note how close you were to what the person identifies as his or her feelings.
- To build empathic rapport, be sure to also ask people to "say more," rather than assume you understand fully what is being expressed.

Ministering Humbly

It is very easy to think that after going to school, getting diplomas, certificates, and licenses, one knows a lot. It is also easy to think that health involves doing the right things and behaving in certain ways. We, ourselves, begin to believe that following the doctor's orders, or the priest's admonitions, will set things right.

To be humble in one's ministry is to try to do your best and help find out what the patient and/or their family feels is right for them. We have no crystal ball. We have experience and ideas that we can share. It is an act of humility to realize that there is a mystery to healing just as there are proven practices. In hospital ministry, we realize that the human spirit and the divine spirit both are the primary cocreators in the healing process. We also realize, with true humility, that there really is a time and a season for everything, including health, illness, life, and death. That realization is truly humbling.

Example

Lorie came to the hospital filled with cancer. This cancer had been working within her for a number of years. The last four years had been particularly challenging. Lorie was a teacher and was determined to live longer than her mother and sister had lived. As fate would have it, she realized that she had lived one year longer than her mother, so far. She was sixty and Labor Day was coming quickly, along with the start of another school year. She wanted to be at home.

She wanted to live. She wanted her family to be optimistic. She believed in the power of positive thinking even though it was difficult for her to put this philosophy into practice. She wanted to live. The chaplain visited her daily and listened to her fears and wishes. She was not very comfortable praying with her family but she could pray with the chaplain. On one occasion she rather angrily asked the chaplain what he believed about her health and her desire to live. The chaplain understood that she wanted to fight to live and that it would be a compassionate thing for him to encourage her to do so. The chaplain also understood that he had no crystal ball and had no idea what God's plan was for Lorie, or how this illness would proceed. With a heavy heart and acknowledgment of the limits of his understanding, the chaplain said, "I only know that we must do the best we can and leave the rest to God." She died in the hospital two weeks later, just after Labor Day.

How to Develop This Skill

- Pray often and pray earnestly "Thy will be done."
- Pay attention to mystery and miracles.
- Reflect on the times when it was a good thing that circumstances did not go the way you thought they would.
- Practice looking for as many options, views, and responses as possible in a given situation.
- Now and again say "I don't know."

MAKING INITIAL CONTACTS

Initial pastoral care contacts have a fairly predictable flow. While each individual may have different styles, the following suggestions would be ideally found in most circumstances. Exceptions would be situations where an emergency is occurring or a specific referral for a specific service has been made.

Planning Ahead

Planning ahead involves making decisions about who to visit, when, and possibly, for what purpose. Planning also involves thinking about available resources should they be needed. If one does not have a sense of the elements involved in making an initial contact, one would need to develop a more concrete plan.

Example

Roberta comes to the office on Friday morning and thinks about what she would like to accomplish the next week. She makes a list and notes any requests or referrals. She responds to those she is able to respond to based on priority. She makes rounds to units C and G. She takes a pen and a note card to write down anything she needs to remember. While making rounds, she speaks with nursing staff to see if there are persons or situations that require attention. She has a regular "spiel" that she uses for most visits.

How to Develop This Skill

- If you tend to need structure, schedule rounds to specific units.
- If you have access to a daily census select a number of persons to visit each day.
- Place all referrals and requests first on your list.
- Decide to visit new admissions or the critically ill.
- Develop a weekly schedule.
- Set aside time to reflect and possibly write out the elements of a visit.
- Notice if there are parts of your initial visits that seem to meet with less than favorable response by you or others.

Showing Up

At some time in hospital ministry, chaplains learn that they cannot be everywhere, and make choices as to where they will go. Because there are so many people to visit, and the task is repetitive, it is quite common to go through periods when it is overwhelming to keep making initial contacts with newly admitted patients. It is, however, a skill, or perhaps a discipline to show up day after day and minister to as many persons as possible.

Example

Rick is in a clinical pastoral education training program in a large city hospital. He is in his seventh week and has managed to demonstrate only fifty hours of pastoral care contacts. He is not sure if he can keep going back. Every day there are new admissions and he isn't sure what to say, whom to visit, or even if he feels like making another visit. He tells all of this to his supervisor who has been in hospital ministry for twenty-five years and often has similar feelings. The supervisor shares this with Rick and says, "we need to keep showing up and doing our job, which is caring for patients."

How to Develop This Skill

- Schedule visits every day.
- Consult regularly with colleagues.
- Place a card beside your computer stating all the reasons you are in hospital ministry. Find other ways to think about what motivates you in this vocation.
- Connect frequently with your mission statement and basic values.

Making Appointments

Making appointments helps with the structuring of daily visitation tasks. These appointments can be quite formal or they can occur less formally during identified times that tend to be good for people. Often, an initial visit needs to be brief. It is often difficult to work around the other treatment processes that also need to occur. Be that as it may, it is crucial to be flexible and willing to catch up with a person after a test, a group, or at another time.

Example

Sara arrives to visit Darlene who is sleeping. Her presence at the door of Darlene's room is just enough for Darlene to move slightly and utter a brief startled noise. Sara decides that today Darlene needs her sleep and that she appears physically comfortable. Softly she says, "You are sleeping. I'll come back."

How to Develop This Skill

- Think of appointments as a courtesy.
- Think of appointments as a way of making choices and getting things done.

- Think of appointments as giving you and the person something to prepare or look forward to doing.
- Carry a card or small appointment book with you as a reminder to make appointments.
- Leave a card or a brochure to let patients know you came by.

Introductions to Patient or Family by Others

Frequently, nurses, nursing assistants, or mental health workers will offer to introduce a patient or family member to the chaplain. At other times, the chaplain may wish to have another staff person make this introduction, or point out the person whom the chaplain intends to visit. Assessing when this introduction would or would not be helpful is a skill.

Example

Father Tom has been asked to provide the Sacrament of the Sick. He realizes that he does not know Sally, who is a patient in the geriatric unit. Rather than fumble around and ask each woman on the unit if she is Sally, he goes directly to the nurse's station and asks for an introduction. The nurse is grateful to be asked, and thankful that she can make a note in the care plan that the sacrament was provided by the priest. Father Tom is able to make three other care visits that afternoon and feels that he has gotten a lot of good work done.

How to Develop This Skill

- When it is appropriate, ask for someone to introduce you to a new patient.
- Be aware of how busy your peers are and the timing of your requests.
- It is an art to be sensitive to discerning what you can do yourself and what you could use help with getting done.

Identifying Yourself and the Services You Provide

Patients and families interact with an amazingly large number of health care professionals. Often these interactions take place in emergency situations and at times when the patient is not as alert or focused as they might be otherwise. It is important to let people know who you are, what you can and cannot do. It is also important to do this professionally and caringly.

Example

Reverend Williams arrived that morning around 10 a.m. He stood behind the nursing station and looked around the unit to see what was happening. He picked up the program booklet to see if there were any new referrals to the loss and recovery group. While standing there, a patient came to the desk and declared that she wanted to see her case manager. Reverend Williams smiled slightly and stated, "I am Chaplain Williams, but I would be glad to ask someone to help you."

How to Develop This Skill

- Observe how other health care professionals introduce themselves.
- In deciding how to introduce yourself, consider what would be the easiest and quickest way for another person to know who you are and what you do.

Timing

There is a rhythm and flow to everything. However, learning that flow and using it to the benefit of self and others takes some practice. Timing in hospital ministry involves knowing when to initiate contacts, what to do when they are interrupted, and knowing when closure makes sense. This kind of flow can be applied to visits as a whole as well as the interactions during visits.

Example

Father Mark arrived on the intensive care unit ready to provide the Sacrament of the Sick. He went straight to the patient's room where he found the curtain drawn around the patient and could hear that there were other persons in the room. He pulled the curtain back only to hear a nurse tell him that this was not a good time. The patient was uncovered and persons were helping attend to her physical needs. Father Mark was insistent, stood where he was, and made no move to leave. The nurse asked him to wait outside. He did not move. In anger and frustration the nurse called on the head chaplain to lodge a complaint. The head chaplain called Father Mark into the office, listened to his account as to what happened, and together they spoke about the issue of timing.

How to Develop This Skill

- If curtains are drawn, other team members are with the patient or family, the patient is asleep, or other cues are present that might indicate bad timing, check with nursing and/or come back later.
- If in doubt, ask.
- When involved with particularly emotionally challenging conversation with a patient, plan to transition to closure at least ten minutes before you are planning to leave.
- Follow the patient's lead as to timing.
- Consider more frequent and brief contacts until physical or mental stability is established

Listening Carefully

Because listening carefully involves so much skill, it is taught in all kinds of people-related settings. In order to listen carefully, one must pay attention to words, look for explicit and implicit meanings, and match words with nonverbal clues. In addition, one must place one's own thoughts on the back burner and focus on the person being listened to. At times, it involves letting the other person know that you are listening and enhancing the process through asking for clarification and expansions of what is being said. The process of listening carefully in hospital ministry also focuses on the search for feelings, meaning, and values, from the perspective of the person doing the talking. Listening carefully can also involve listening for what is not being said.

Example

A number of years ago the Protestant and Catholic chaplains were conducting a joint service on admissions. This involved both a Mass and a Protestant Communion. One homily was preached and there was one pastoral prayer. The chaplains took turns. On this particular Sunday, the Protestant chaplain was leading the prayers and asked for prayer concerns. A middle-aged man said that "his dog had died," and went on with a description about what happened. When it came time for the pastoral prayer, the chaplain prayed about the dog that had died and the sadness of its owner. In the midst of this, the man spoke up and declared, at the top of his voice, "No, I didn't say my dog had died; I said the police shot my dog." Needless to say, the chaplain thought about her listening skills!

How to Develop This Skill

- Find a resource that breaks down the skill of listening into behavioral parts.
- Check occasionally to find out if you are hearing correctly— You might ask, "Are you saying. . . ."
- After a visit, write down what the person said and see if you can recover the main points, the feeling tone, things that might have been omitted and the meaning put forth in the conversation.
- Be sure to establish eye contact, if possible, and put on hold any things that you are thinking or feeling that could be distracting to the process of listening.
- View every initial contact as a time to gather important information helpful to providing quality and meaningful ministry.

Reflections on Outcomes of Visit

Every contact has an outcome. By outcome, one is referring to some kind of change. The desired outcomes for initial visits/contacts with patients are gathering information, introduction of self and services, being supportive, if possible, and assessing how to be of further help with particular attention given to spiritual and holistic health care and recovery.

Example

A clinical pastoral intern reflects at the end of a visit, "Throughout the visit, I wasn't sure if I was connecting with the family member. I think I was a pleasant and supportive presence, but I do not think that I reflected some of the feelings of shock and loss that the person was feeling."

How to Develop This Skill

- Develop a plan with a decision tree format to use with initial contacts. This way you can have several ways to proceed depending on what happens.
- Think of the contact as being 20 percent yours and 80 percent the patients'.
- Ask patients what they would like to have happen.
- After a contact, think about what happened and whether there is more to do.
- Remember that outcomes can not all be identified immediately.
- Outcomes are behavioral and observable but not always immediate.

PROVIDING PRACTICAL HELP

Focusing

To be helpful to a patient, one must first focus on the patient. This sounds a bit simplistic, but problems with focus can become a stumbling block at any point in the practice of hospital ministry. By focus I refer to the skill of bringing full attention to the patient and his or her needs. This is really the most important way to be truly helpful. Failure to do this well often results in providing inadequate help. Conversely, doing it well leads to individualized services that can promote health and healing.

Example

The chaplain was visiting the mother of a child in pediatrics. The visit was pleasant and lasted about fifteen minutes. The mother admitted to being tired. Yet, throughout the conversation, she kept a watchful eye on her child. The conversation included telling the chaplain about the child's illness. The mother also talked about some of her fears. She told the chaplain that she was Catholic. At the end of the time, the chaplain offered to pray for the family. This was well received. However, when the chaplain started to pray, the mother was surprised and said so. After some discussion, the mother agreed to have the chaplain pray at that time. The chaplain later had difficulty remembering anything that the mother had said. The chaplain left feeling quite tired and began thinking of his growing list of things to do.

How to Develop This Skill

- Make notes about a contact immediately after the contact.
- Consider what makes this person's story unique.
- Try to remember one to two themes only and one to two predominant feelings expressed.
- Go back for a follow-up visit.
- Pay attention to information that may need to be filled-in by the patient.
- Be able to answer the question as to what would be helpful or not helpful.

Sorting

For many reasons a hospitalized person may have difficulty focusing on their needs and situation, and may have difficulty sorting through what is going on inside. It can be very helpful to have a chaplain available to spend time helping them focus on what is happening. It can also be very helpful to have a chaplain help them sort through their thoughts, and feelings, and identify needs. Often, these needs are in addition to the physical care needs that are being addressed by other health care providers.

Sorting is a skill that a chaplain can use with patients who are particularly overwhelmed. By giving the patient undivided attention, the chaplain is able to hear some of the issues that are perhaps not being attended to, or that properly belong to the realm of spiritual care and spiritual healing. In many cases where there is spiritual distress and complexity of health care issues, the chaplain can be of great help in assisting the patient as he or she makes initial choices on the path to recovery.

Example

Mildred had been in the hospital for some time. As she thought about the things that were happening while she was in the hospital, her anxiety and depression grew. When she turned her thoughts to her health and recovery and the length of her hospitalization, she was equally overwhelmed. Finally she made an appointment with the chaplain saying, "I want to see if I can sort this out and make some sense of all this." As it turned out, they had to meet several times before Mildred and the chaplain could sort enough to come up with a plan for focusing on the most important things Mildred felt she had to process.

How to Develop This Skill

- Teach yourself a system for sorting. Use a system you can easily teach to patients.
- Your system for sorting may not be helpful to a patient due to their individual style. Find out how patients work on problem solving when they are feeling well.

Referring

The skill of referring and receiving referrals is based on the reasoning that not everyone can meet every patient need. Good referrals are based on reasonably accurate assessments of what would be helpful to the patient and on who is able to provide that service. The second part of the skill of referring, or receiving referrals, is a sound sense of one's own skills and limitations. Referrals in the field of hospital ministry could go to the department, to a specific chaplain, to a consultant within the hospital, or to someone in the larger faith community. Of course, referrals for pastoral care and counseling are received predominantly from nurses, doctors, social services, psychology departments, treatment teams, families, and friends.

Example

The chaplain received a call from the charge nurse on the day shift. The nurse was concerned about a decidedly downward shift in the physical functioning of a patient on her unit. Not only was the cancer advancing at a rapid rate, but the patient appeared to be getting more and more withdrawn and depressed. The nurse was aware that there might be nothing anyone could do to save this patient's life. Still, she hoped that a visit from the chaplain might help with the growing despair the patient was experiencing. The chaplain listened to the referral for services and remembered that a colleague had a productive care visit with this person the last time she was hospitalized. He picked up the phone and made a referral to his colleague.

How to Develop This Skill

- When a referral is made, consider the service requested and think about the best person to provide that service.
- When you are the only chaplain available, consider whether or not to bring in a consultant.
- If you need to provide the service requested, and don't feel very comfortable, consult with a colleague or find other resources to help you prepare to provide the service.
- Practice making referrals to persons in other disciplines.
- Learn about how other disciplines/departments make referrals.

Advocacy

In a sense, every member of the health care team/organization is a patient advocate. It is everyone's responsibility to pay attention to patient's rights and the hospital's responsibilities. The hospital ministry department has an additional role of being supportive to religious and spiritual care rights and of being aware of ethical issues. In a less formal sense, it is part of the chaplain's role to help empower patients in their recovery. Often this can be done by helping patients focus and sort through their thoughts, feelings, and experiences, and then refer them to persons who could be helpful. Occasionally, the chaplain will need to speak to others on behalf of the patient. When this is the case, every effort should be made to get the help needed in an appropriate and timely manner. At the same time, it is important to support the team in their work at providing quality health care.

Example

Sandra came into the hospital in an agitated state. She did not want to be there. She felt that her rights had been violated by the revocation of her conditional discharge. During past hospitalizations, she benefitted from attending chapel services. However, nursing felt that this was not a time to take her to the chapel service, so her request was declined. This went on for several weeks. Sandra finally contacted the chaplain and complained. The chaplain understood why the team had refused to give Sandra privileges and yet also knew that Sandra usually benefitted from attending chapel services. In fact, chapel services appeared to be therapeutic for Sandra and helped with her behavior after the service. Usually, the chaplain did not intervene, preferring that Sandra take responsibility for her own behavior. However, this time the chaplain spoke with nursing on Sandra's behalf and was able to negotiate a plan for getting her to and from services the following Sunday. This was all contingent on Sandra's behavior during the week. The plan was reviewed with Sandra who saw it as a hopeful sign and something to work for during the days ahead. The chaplain felt good about advocating for a patient's right in a way that was collegial and respectful of everyone and therapeutic for the patient.

How to Develop This Skill

- Learn about the rights of patients in your hospital.
- Learn about complaint procedures.
- Focus in particular about patients religious rights and determine the specific response that would be applied in your hospital situation.
- At each opportunity, consider how or if you can be helpful. Apply the adage of "do no harm" to your considerations.
- Always consider first how the patient can be empowered.

Resources

Health care chaplains are faced with the task of knowing about a variety of religious and spiritual care resources. These resources are often tangible items that the pastoral care department has on hand or knows how to get. In addition to internal department resources, the chaplain has an obligation to know the health care system and hospital well enough to access other resources.

Example

On Monday morning Tom requested a copy of the Koran by filling out the chaplain's request form. Becky wanted a copy of *These Days,* and Olivia had heard of the book of prayers that the chaplain's department had placed in the chapel. Georgette wanted a rosary before going to court, and Chet thought it would be nice to have one of those

Celtic crosses since he had given the previous one to a friend who was having a difficult evening. Ken chimed in a request for a King James Bible as the chaplain passed by. The morning was busy and thank goodness all the items were available in the office and could be brought to people later in the afternoon. However, another Koran would need to be obtained to have as back up since this one was a department loaner.

How to Develop This Skill

- Develop a budget for purchasing basic crosses, rosaries, devotional guides.
- Develop a relationship with the Bible Society and the Gideons who often provide Bibles free of cost.
- Consider getting Care Notes and other material specific to hospital spiritual care.
- Visit and/or call other hospitals to find out what resources they use.
- Consider having a chaplain request form.

Spiritual Care Practices

Sometimes chaplains focus on just two or three spiritual care practices. These practices usually include: saying prayers, reading the Bible, and administering sacraments or other rites. However, in today's world of increasing plurality of beliefs and nonreligious spiritual care practices, one has to develop skill in other practices. To meet these needs, it is important to consider spiritual care practices that can be used in the hospital setting as well as skills that can be used after the patient leaves the hospital. Practices that can be used in the future can be considered part of spiritual care discharge planning.

Example

Kathy was quite anxious about the forthcoming procedure. It was only a biopsy of her breast. Still, it had been very scary to see the dark spot on the mammogram and to feel the lump the size of her thumbnail. She came to the hospital an hour early, but was so anxious and teary-eyed that the worker who checked her in felt it would be helpful to call the hospital chaplain, who was friendly and seemed to have helped other patients in the past. Chaplain Jones came as soon as she received the page. She introduced herself to Kathy and asked if she could sit down. Kathy talked about her fears and indicated that she just couldn't manage them. She indicated that she wasn't very religious. Chaplain Jones asked if Kathy had any favorite saying that she used to help her get through difficult times. Kathy thought for a bit and remembered the saying, "This too shall pass." It was a saying her grandmother had always said when Kathy faced disappointment or any other kind of problem. The chaplain thought this was a fine saying and suggested they say it together a few times. "If need be," the chaplain declared, "you can think of another wise saying after you get through this step." Kathy spent the rest of the time on her own. As she waited, she repeated the little phrase over and over again.

How to Develop This Skill

- Keep an ongoing list of spiritual practices as you discover them.
- Ask patients what spiritual practices they use.
- Learn new practices such as deep breathing, brief meditations, use of mantras, journaling, and the reading of uplifting literature.

Use of Prayers

One of the ways that a chaplain can be of practical help is through the use of prayer. Of course, it is a skill and an art to know how and when to use prayers, and to what purpose. In recent years, much research has demonstrated the efficacy of prayers. This research has convincingly shown some that prayer can be helpful to people whether or not they know they are being prayed for. Recently, Larry Dossey (1993) has indicated that prayers in a negative spirit may also increase the possibility of negative effects. In fact, he admonishes us to be careful what we pray for, and to be careful in asking people to pray for us!

Example

Kelly found herself in dialysis for the third time in one week, and she was so discouraged that she found herself praying aloud. "Dear God," she prayed, " I know you helped my mother when she faced cancer. I prayed to you to let her live and she lived a long and healthy life. They say I need a kidney soon and I know you will help me if you can. Thanks. Amen." Kelly felt silly asking for a kidney so straight-forwardly but she just knew that prayers worked somehow. A week later a kidney was available and Kelly received one. Some of her friends said that the kidney was available because of coincidence and aided by the fact that Kelly's name was next on the list. Kelly believed that it was a miracle and that her prayers were answered. She knew that all her prayers hadn't been answered so grandly or obviously through the years. Still, she was glad that this one was answered so quickly and she thanked God right away.

How to Develop This Skill

- Set aside time to pray daily.
- Learn about the different functions of prayers.
- Learn prayers from a variety of sacred sources.
- Encourage patients to pray for themselves as they are able.
- Mention prayer as a spiritual practice and teach patients how to pray simply and directly.
- List the prayer resources available in your ministry.
- Provide places for prayer.
- Use the conversational technique of saying out loud what you would say to God.
- When you say you will pray for someone, or keep them on your prayer list, do so within a few minutes of the visit so that you will not forget.

Use of Scripture or Sacred Texts

It is especially common for conservative religious students to feel that they have not completed a pastoral care visit without bringing the person to Christ. They struggle with persons of differing reli-gions including persons who are Christian but of a differing faith group. Hence, they are often caught between their profound beliefs and learning skills of ministering to persons who do not believe as they do. The skill of knowing how people choose and use sacred texts is crucial to chaplains in hospital ministry. So, too, is the knowledge of when scripture, or sacred texts, are and likely to be healing.

Example

Barry was dressed in a black T-shirt with all kinds of skulls and crossbones. He usually dressed this way. This afternoon he noted that the chaplain's door was open so he dropped in to ask if the chaplain knew anything about warlocks, animal powers, and witchcraft. He said that he believed in these things and wanted to learn more. Admittedly, the chaplain silently wondered about how much of Barry's interests were due to his psychosis, and how much were part of his belief system. However, the chaplain chose to take the request straightforwardly and suggested that Barry look these things up in the public library or in a large bookstore when he had the opportunity back home. The chaplain could tell that Barry appreciated this direct answer as evidenced by his hearty "thank you" upon leaving the office.

How to Develop This Skill

- Ask the patient if he or she has favorite "readings" from his or her tradition.
- Ask if any of these would be helpful at this time.
- Read from different traditions for the purposes of understanding and providing care to those who believe differently than you do.
- Feel free to wonder respectfully about readings that are perhaps being used in what you wonder is a healthy or healing way.

SUPPORTIVE STRATEGIES

Supportive strategies can be found in all of the practical helps listed in the preceding example. They are a part of the relational approach that forms a thread running through all quality pastoral care services. In order for any care intervention to be supportive, it must meet the requirement of emotionally holding the patient in a caring way. Whenever the patient feels cared for, the patient feels supported. This makes it very challenging to be supportive, since the perception of supportiveness resides with the recipient and not with the care provider's intention. There are limits to being supportive, and when these limits are reached, the chaplain may need to move into brief counseling, making a referral, or back to strategies mentioned previously in this chapter.

It is not necessarily supportive to just listen and agree with a person. Patients who are ambivalent will see right through this. When this happens it is likely that an initial experience of support may later be found to be seriously wanting. To be supportive, one must first listen, try to understand, and find out what the individual is thinking, feeling, and perhaps planning.

Understand before being understood.

Steven Covey lists this as a habit of effective people, in other words, one might use the adage, "know thyself" and then "support others." Covey speaks of empathic listening which leads to deep understanding. "When we really, deeply understand each other, we open the door to creative solutions and third alternatives. Our differences are no longer stumbling blocks to communication and progress. Instead, they become the stepping stones to synergy" (Covey, 1990, p. 259).

Support persons who may not be easy to support.

You don't have to like a person to support that person. Remember, down the road you will find that some of the patients who were the most resistant and challenging may become those who have traveled the longest way toward health and healing. When it is not easy to support a person, think of where the barriers or obstacles to support might be. Brainstorm what must happen to make support easier. If you can't be supportive, and the person cannot give you help as to what would feel supportive, consider the possibility that what is needed may not be support, but counseling. Also, consider that barriers may lie within you, and may be due to what is stirred up by relating to the person. If this might be the issue, you may need to make a referral, or get some help working through your own thoughts and feelings. Never support anything that is destructive to the patient or to others. That is not real support and is quite dangerous for everyone involved.

Admit when you are trying to be supportive but are finding it difficult.

There is a saying in the counseling field that when there is a giraffe (or huge problem) in the room it is a good idea to name the giraffe or problem. To keep trying to be supportive and having it fail will only make the relationship stuck, and thus thwart healing possibilities. It is important to recognize failures to be supportive without assigning blame. If the problem is with the care provider, then reflection on that problem is better accomplished at another time. Instead, consider asking the patient what he or she would find helpful. Learning what the patient finds supportive is a basic pastoral care question. So, too, is the question of how one can be supportive. Significant difficulties in identifying and receiving support may have to be left for counseling efforts that may focus on the underlying causes of this dynamic.

Accept all feelings and thoughts but not necessarily behaviors.

Remember that people value their thoughts and feelings even when they don't like that fact that they have them. However, thoughts and feelings are value neutral for chaplains. Therefore, all thoughts and feelings can, and should be, heard in a supportive or listening way. However, any thoughts or feelings that could turn into inappropriate behavior should be discussed and perhaps confronted. Necessary confrontations can vary in technique and intensity depending on the concern identified.

Help people name any feelings that they may struggle with.

Don't gloss over feelings such as anger, fear, or loneliness. But, don't necessarily dig deeper either. Just help them be noticed as feelings. When possible, encourage the person to name his or her feelings. Follow up the naming of a feeling being experienced with a brief query as to whether there are other feelings. Often, it may be necessary and helpful for the chaplain to name a few possible feelings just to get the process going.

Recognize that denial is a protective coating and is present for a reason.

If you need to let a person know that he or she is in denial, do so in a very normative way. You might say that we all use denial to protect ourselves during difficult times. It's natural. However, if you bring up denial, be prepared to state what the person did, or said, that caused you to think that the denial mechanism was being used. Never suggest that the person abandon this denial, even if it is a gross misperception of reality. If you feel you have a good relationship with the patient, you may choose to gently wonder about the person's thinking or beliefs. You may also let the conversation drop, follow up at another time, and/or consult with a colleague.

Recognize that many people feel conflicted about their beliefs and faith traditions, and about chaplains and spiritual care.

Taking a neutral and nondefensive stance can be very supportive. Recognize that you do not need to defend anything or any belief. Often, taking a slightly curious or interested approach can be very helpful as well as supportive.

There is always more than one way to be supportive; if one way doesn't work, look for another.

Remember that you can be indirectly supportive of someone who declines your services. You may, for example, work with teams and team members, you may refer to colleagues, you may let the situation sit for a bit, you may offer it up in prayer. Tell yourself that there are at least three ways to be supportive in any given situation. Follow this by making a mental list of these three ways no matter how rational. In some cases, it might be a good idea to get a particularly challenging patient to come up with three ways that they feel would be supportive to them. Often, patients can tell you what has to happen for them to be supported.

BRIEF COUNSELING

When supportive strategies have reached their limits and more focused and skilled pastoral care is needed, it may indicate the need for brief pastoral/spiritual care counseling. This may mean that a referral to other resources within the hospital is in order, or that follow-up pastoral counseling services be recommended. It may also mean a movement of pastoral care services back to earlier processes such as occasional contact and practical help. Brief counseling in hospital ministry is usually provided for patients, family, and other employees.

Beginnings

It is very important to identify the time when one moves from supportive care to brief counseling. In its less rigorous sense, this would be the moment when the chaplain or spiritual care provider identifies a problem and begins to work on helping the person work through that problem. In a hospital setting there are many occasions for counseling. Some of these occasions come at first contact as part of a crisis in health care, or on occasions when one is planning to provide practical help. Regardless of how smooth or abrupt the transition from support to counseling, the process, once started, is quite different due to the nature of the goals, interventions, and identification of expected completion such as discharge or referral.

Example

Theresa came to the hospital to deliver her first child. The delivery went well, and Theresa and the baby appeared to be fine. However, the nurse noticed that Theresa was sad and she could not get Theresa to talk about her thoughts and feelings. The nurse called the chaplain and asked him if he would visit Theresa. Theresa shared with the chaplain that the baby was not her husband's, and that she was feeling guilty and scared about what would happen should her husband find out. The complexity of the situation caused the chaplain to realize that a much more focused process was needed, and began to internally formulate a brief treatment plan that could be initiated while Theresa was still in the hospital, which would conclude with referral strategies for further counseling. Since Theresa and her baby would only spend two days in the hospital, the chaplain spent forty-five minutes with Theresa and made an appointment for a second session the next day. They both agreed that they would focus on two things: expression of her thoughts and feelings and developing a plan for what she wanted to happen.

How to Develop This Skill

- Consider brief counseling as a "piece of the work," not the whole process.

- Consider the following factors: the initiator of the counseling, the relationship, the location, time available, purpose of the counseling.
- Practice identifying moments when you are being supportive and helpful and moments when you are working hard to help a patient through a process or issue.
- At the point of deciding to begin counseling, also establish a point of ending so that you can keep focused and develop a true treatment plan.
- Read and take courses on brief counseling.

Presenting Problem

A presenting problem that indicates a possible need for brief counseling is something that is acute (has symptoms that are currently overwhelming or unmanageable and require quick relief) or something that by its nature needs to be addressed for health and healing to occur. Presenting problems are usually prioritized according to their perceived risk to stabilization, health, and safety. Presenting problems are things considered problematic from the patient's point of view. However, there are patients who are not able to identify some of the problems that interfere with treatment, health, and healing. In some cases, the presenting problem is considered problematic from the referral source's point of view. Thus, the presenting problem may be identified through the assessment processes of the pastoral health care provider. While clinical pastoral interns are taught to focus on the patient's identified problem, the presenting problem which brings a person to pastoral care or counseling may come from many sources in practice. For a list of typical presenting problems that may lend themselves to brief counseling, consult Appendix O.

Example

Julie was brought to the psychiatric ward in a defiant and angry mood. She felt she should be able to kill herself if she wanted. She blamed her family and doctor for putting her in the hospital, saying that nothing she had done was so problematic that she should be confined for treatment. She was assigned to the loss and recovery group because she had recently lost custody of her child. She refused to talk in the group, saying that she had no losses, and that it wasn't anyone's business.

How to Develop This Skill

- Every time contact is made with a patient, make a mental list of what the person states, implicitly or explicitly, as his or her problems.
- Practice categorizing problems that come up in the categories of urgent, important, and can be handled later.
- Consider who to refer urgent problems to if you decide not to focus on those problems yourself.
- Consider how long the person will be hospitalized before you work on important problems. If you go into these areas, do so after urgent problems are processed.
- Place an imaginary hold sign on problems "to be handled later" and suggest to that patient that these be placed on hold for now, but may be followed up at a later date.
- Consult with another peer about items you have deemed urgent.

Treatment Goals

Brief counseling in the hospital setting is usually solution-focused and/or promotes symptom reduction. In either case, the expression of thoughts and feelings is considered helpful. Occasionally, a person who is having difficulty thinking, and having less difficulty expressing feelings, will be encouraged to state his or her thoughts. Conversely, a person who thinks a lot may be encouraged to identify possible feelings that go along with his or her thoughts. In any case, the treatment goals for brief counseling are modest. Treatment goals are also best stated in behavioral terms so that the chaplain or pastoral counselor and the patient and/or family can have confidence about the changes sought. Some possible goals are:

- To process options for treatment and to make choices
- To express feelings about what is happening
- To talk about how one perceives God or a higher power being involved
- To manage the beginning stages of grieving

- To identify and process relationships sufficiently to reduce current acute symptoms such as refusal of treatment, self-harming thoughts, upcoming court happenings, or functioning on the job (for hospital employees)

Example

Henry came to work on Tuesday and was feeling okay about his job at the hospital. The day was filled with activity, and Henry liked it that way. However, at 2:00 in the afternoon, Henry was moved to another unit. As he was walking down the hall, a patient came up to him and out of the blue, socked him in the jaw, then kicked him while he was on the floor. Henry was given immediate care and luckily, nothing was broken. However, he was badly shaken up and had difficulty going back on the unit. His supervisor suggested that Henry speak with someone from the employee assistance department, but Henry was reluctant to do so. The supervisor then suggested that Henry speak with one of the chaplains. Henry agreed, and made an appointment for that afternoon. Because this was such a traumatic event, the chaplain and Henry ended up meeting once a week for four weeks. At the end of that time, both agreed that Henry had processed what had happened and how he was feeling about it. His anxiety was reduced enough to be considered a "healthy alertness" to what was happening around him. He agreed to take a brush-up in-service course on cues to managing aggressive behavior. He also agreed to call if he felt he needed further help.

How to Develop This Skill

- Learn to identify symptoms relating to identified problems.
- Find a good book about solution focused counseling.
- Involve yourself in continuing education efforts around problem areas that you are most likely to find in your setting.

Treatment Interventions

Brief counseling treatment interventions for acute care hospital ministry are designed to help the patient cope in the present and work through obstacles toward healing and recovery issues. For some of this to happen, the patient may have to process some material from the past. But, the reason for doing so is for relating to present health, illness, and recovery issues. As a rule of thumb, it is wise to use feeling words and phrases when helping the patient express his or her feelings. That would mean using thinking-type phrases when helping with problems of processing at the thinking level. Do not let the patient regress into unmanageable material.

For the purposes of brief counseling and rapid stabilization and recovery, it is helpful to listen actively and focus on phrases that suggest functioning and management of thoughts and feelings. Reframing thoughts and feelings in a more positive and hopeful light can work very well as long as it is not outrageously different than what would fit with facts from the patient's perspective. Spiritual care practices that tend to be helpful in brief counseling are those that help the patient feel more hopeful, more loved, and possibly aided by God or a higher power.

Remember, in hospital ministry you may only see a person once. Due to circumstances beyond your control, the person may be discharged. Therefore, the final part of any brief counseling session must always end with some type of summary. This summary would ideally pull together thoughts and feelings, problems and progress, and plans no matter how incomplete.

Example

Matthew was quite angry with his mother for what he felt was her siding with the doctors in insisting that he be hospitalized. He had made several suicidal attempts. He talked quite openly in his first session with a pastoral counseling intern. The intern noticed that his predominant feeling was anger, and that he used violent self-harming attempts to commit suicide. The intern knew that it was highly possible that Matthew might someday succeed in killing himself. She desperately tried to think of an intervention that might change that rapid movement from thoughts to anger to action. Quite softly, she said to Matthew, "You know I've heard people admit that they often are the angriest at persons they care the most about." There was a long pause in the conversation and Matthew went on to talk about his beliefs and recounted other experiences that did not relate to his anger. The pastoral counseling intern came to supervision feeling that she had at least tried something.

How to Develop This Skill

- Develop a typical process for brief counseling.
- To develop this process, review typical experiences you have had or that you find through other resources.
- In reviewing brief counseling sessions, practice considering several interventions. Think through how each intervention could be used to accomplish different things.
- Have handy guidelines for brief pastoral counseling goals and interventions.

Endings

In hospital ministry, there is not always a crisp beginning and ending to counseling. Therefore, it is crucial to see each session as somewhat independent of other sessions, unless you have information that proves otherwise. However, this does not mean that a one-time pastoral counseling session reverts to becoming supportive, or that it focuses on spiritual care practices and resources. As stated earlier, counseling is distinguished from general care techniques by the focused assessment, diagnosis, goal setting, and treatment plan with counseling interventions. You may end the counseling process as soon as you and the patient agree that you have finished. Endings must convey the completion of counseling work and the changing of the relationship, if that is the case.

Example

Earl was having difficulty with the news that he had cancer and that it had invaded many of his internal organs and systems. He was only forty-two and totally unprepared for what might be difficult and greatly shortened final days. He was quite ill, and intensely grieving. Earl's doctor was in bright and early on a Monday morning to talk with him. The doctor felt that it would be helpful for Earl to have someone to help him through the grieving process so that things would not get too complicated. The doctor thought immediately of the chaplain who served on the medical ethics committee. She knew that the chaplain was also a licensed pastoral psychotherapist and thought this would be a good match. Due to the crisis in time, the chaplain decided to meet with Earl daily. They met four times that week, and both felt that it had been helpful. Earl was assured that the chaplain would stop in to check on him, and should Earl go home, he could feel free to call the chaplain. Earl decided that he might choose the services of hospice, and thought that if he did so he would likely seek the services of the hospice chaplain as well as the minister of his church.

How to Develop This Skill

- Begin by reflecting on how you feel about endings. Pay particular attention to your preferred style.
- After consulting brief counseling methods, make note of what are considered standards for terminating counseling.
- Consider endings as part of the counseling process.
- Always ask patients for feedback about the counseling process and how they prefer to end counseling.

CRISIS MINISTRY

Crisis ministry, a specialized and complex ministry, involves advanced pastoral skills. It is included in this chapter because a crisis event can happen as early as day one of a new ministry. For purposes of this chapter, one will assume that an entry level chaplain will need to at least provide the equivalent of spiritual care "first aid" by drawing on skills mentioned under common sense, initial contacts, practical helps, support, and even brief counseling. In addition, there is a need to know the basic elements of a crisis situation, as well as generic, helpful responses.

Preparation and Practice for Crisis Ministry

While practice is a form of preparation, it is often done in noncritical moments for the purposes of learning. Preparation for the management of crises usually involves documentation of these processes in the form of written procedures, protocols, policies, and competencies. Crises managed by pastoral care staff include hospitalwide crises, unit-specific crises, and person-specific crises. The on call or emergency availability of the pastoral care department may include specific response guidelines that serve as expectations during moments of crisis. Knowledge about the clinical pastoral elements of crisis interventions are best learned through specialized continuing education opportunities.

Example

In September, the hospital asked every department to review its procedures for evacuating disabled persons. It occurred to the pastoral services department that such an occurrence might happen on a Sunday morning during worship services in the hospital. They realized that they not only had no plan, they had no idea what to do. A chaplain met with the hospital's safety manager and devised a safety management plan. The process was initiated soon thereafter.

How to Develop This Skill

- Take clinical pastoral training units that include opportunities to practice responding to crisis.
- Gather resources on crisis ministry.
- Work with other departments concerning crises that affect the hospital as a whole.
- Develop a specific protocol for how the hospital ministry will respond to various crises.

Assessment of Crisis Ministry Events

Crisis ministry is a response to an event that has life-threatening potential. It may include experiences of emotional, spiritual, physical, and social trauma. Crisis itself is a moment considered atypical of ordinary functioning. It is usually unwanted, and the person(s) experiencing it are usually unprepared.

Crisis ministry includes responses to challenging births where a new life might be threatened. It includes responses to persons in intense pain, or who are experiencing fear, anxiety, and/or may be dying. It also includes emotional and spiritual instances of intense pain. A crisis may indeed be the pervasive "dark night of the soul."

Crises may include times when information is presented to patients that will likely require supportive endeavors. Crises are always assessed as to degree of risk to health or safety, intensity of internal suffering, and the potential for a pastoral intervention to be the type of intervention that would decrease risk and suffering.

Example

Baby Jody's mother and father brought her to the hospital. She had been found underwater in the family's small wading pool. It was quite possible that Jody would never recover. While the treatment team worked with Jody, the nurse felt it was a good idea to call the chaplain to be with the parents. The chaplain was paged, using the hospital's arranged system for such emergencies. The chaplain on-call came immediately.

How to Develop This Skill

- Gather information from experienced chaplains as to what they believe constitutes crises and how they assess crises.
- Develop criteria of your own about what you consider a crisis in your setting.
- Whenever you are faced with a new crisis, take time to reflect later on how you determined what constituted the crisis.
- Have informal or formal departmental reviews of all crises after they occur.

Interventions During Crisis Events

Interventions are a chaplain's behaviors during a crises event. Some crises will follow hospitalwide standard procedures. Crises on the unit that do not involve pastoral care specifically, may sometimes benefit from the help of a nearby chaplain. Often, this type of help includes supporting other patients or standing near the nursing station as a calming presence. Other than these interventions, do not do anything that you have not been asked or trained to do.

A possible reminder of intervening in a crisis where you have been asked to provide specific crisis ministry services is to use the acronym REASSURE:

R: **respond** immediately
E: **enter** the situation carefully
A: **assess** for risk to person(s) and self

S: **stabilize** the situation as quickly and as calmly as possible
S: **support** the person in a calming manner
U: **understand** the source of the crisis
R: **resource** helpful actions or interventions with patient
E: **evaluate** further needs

Example

Debbie was admitted to the hospital having been dragged from a cult group by her concerned parents. She was young and showed symptoms of post-traumatic stress disorder that included psychotic material. At present she was in seclusion. When asked about what would be helpful, she said that she would like to see a minister. The chaplain was called. The chaplain spoke with the head nurse and with Debbie's mental health workers before deciding to enter the seclusion room where Debbie was. The chaplain was told that Debbie was not assaultive. The chaplain presented a calming presence using tone of voice and posture. Debbie sat on a mat on the floor. After a few minutes, the chaplain asked if she could sit on the floor, across the room from Debbie. The chaplain listened to Debbie talk about her experiences and tried to understand what was happening. She asked Debbie what would be helpful, and was told that it was a matter of life and death that the chaplain pray for her soul. Debbie felt that she needed this prayer throughout the day. The chaplain offered to pray with her, and that offer was accepted. Furthermore, the chaplain explained to Debbie that she kept a daily prayer list and would add her name to that list. She seemed momentarily hopeful, laid on the mat, and turned her face toward the wall. The chaplain left.

How to Develop This Skill

- Do what you need to do to develop a crisis intervention process that you can mange in most situations.
- Reflect and consult periodically about crisis interventions with colleagues and peers.

Follow-Up After a Crisis Event

It is not always possible, or necessary, to follow up on a crisis event. This sounds at first glance like a controversial stance. However, in the practice of hospital ministry, there is a certain practicality and priority of services that must be maintained. To this end, certain rules of thumb apply. The first rule is if you say you are going to come back, then you need to come back. If you suggest that you are available if needed, and indicate how the person may contact you, it becomes the person's choice to initiate that contact. If you are in the habit of making rounds, checking in with a patient or a member of their treatment team makes sense. If the circumstances of a crisis dictate the usual and customary practice of providing a specific service, such as counseling, then the follow-up is essential. Generally follow-ups to crisis are initiated within the next working day.

Example

Ren was in the substance abuse treatment program when he heard that his wife had left him for someone else. He was beside himself and convinced that he had not seen this coming. Somehow, he was able to obtain some alcohol and while drunk tried to harm himself. As soon as his vital signs had stabilized, he threatened to hurt himself again, or someone else, if he did not see the priest right away. The on-call priest was asked to come in and did so. After about thirty minutes, Ren calmed down and fell asleep. The priest decided that the situation warranted a follow-up visit, and possibly a referral for pastoral counseling. So, he came back the next day to talk while Ren was sober.

How to Develop This Skill

- Follow-up skills involve prioritization of care and practices of organized scheduling.
- Each time you conduct a follow-up meeting, decide the goal of the contact.

Evaluating the Crisis Event and Receiving Feedback

Every crisis event warrants a special occurrence review, no matter whether it is conducted formally or informally. The process of evaluating the event, and receiving feedback as to interventions and outcomes, is helpful to the provision of services, everyone's learning, and professional/personal growth.

Example

After the priest in the preceding example met with Ren, he followed up with a visit the next day. He asked Ren what helped, and what did not help. The priest also asked the attending nurse about her impressions of the event, and finally, the priest consulted with the other chaplain in the department of pastoral care. Not everyone saw the situation in the same light, but the priest felt he had learned something that would help him the next time an event like this happened.

How to Develop This Skill

- During the practicing stages of learning to follow up and receive feedback after a crisis, prepare a journal entry or process note or form for structuring your feedback.
- Evaluate your response to the crisis using criteria that you can check on a scale of 1 to 5.
- After an event consider asking yourself the question, "How can I improve?"

In summary, it is not unusual for a seminarian to be engaged in parish ministry having had approximately ten weeks of clinical training in a hospital setting. Nor is it unusual for colleagues in health care to underestimate the extent of training that goes into becoming a skilled chaplain. However, those who have worked in this field know that one is never completely at ease with one's skills and responses to the challenging situations found in every hospital setting. For these reasons, it is crucial that we talk about and share information concerning the skills needed to do the work we do. Besides, being good at what we do helps everyone.

Chapter 8

Going Beyond the Basics

God does not seem to want leaders to "settle" for a little piece of land, spiritual or otherwise. The Divine constantly urges us to lift up our eyes and see all the possibilities on the horizon and to shake off the dust and ashes from our minds and feet and get going. (Jones, 1995, p. 109)

While chaplains are expected to be able to function using the skills mentioned in the previous chapter, it is quite common for individual chaplains to wish to advance professionally. Therefore, in this chapter, we will explore eight areas in which a chaplain may wish to specialize:

1. Administrative skills and functions
2. Consultation
3. Biomedical and professional ethics
4. Advanced pastoral care
5. Advanced pastoral counseling
6. Training programs, supervision, and teaching
7. Contributions to the field—research and writing
8. Interpretation and advocacy within the wider community

In many cases, a chaplain will specialize in several areas. In some cases, chaplains will limit themselves to direct pastoral care, pastoral care with a specific age group, or to a specific health care field, such as pediatrics. When specialization occurs, the chaplain is said to have developed, formally or informally, a competency in that particular field or area of hospital ministry.

MAKING USE OF THIS CHAPTER

This chapter can be helpful to the reader in a number of ways. You may decide to:

- Assess your personal/professional ministry and development.
- Identify areas for advancement and specialization.
- Devise a personal plan for professional development.
- Use the information to generate a mission and vision for your pastoral care department.
- Use the information in the selection of future staff.
- Use this information to interpret the focus and content of your ministry for your supervisor and/or organization.

ADMINISTRATIVE SKILLS AND FUNCTIONS

Administrative advancement within the field of hospital ministry is usually accomplished through two modes. The first is a move to supervisory level functioning, and the second is a move to management functions. In both cases, the person is usually directing other chaplains, consultants, and possibly volunteers. Additional administrative modes include generalized leadership and broader spiritual care leadership functions. The following leadership modes may occur within the pastoral care department or within the organization at advanced levels:

- Supervision
- Administrative skills
- Leadership
- Spiritual care leadership

Supervision Within the Organization

While chaplains frequently find themselves in supervisory roles early in their ministry, they do not necessarily have training and skills in organizational supervision. If they have received training, it has more than likely been in supervising students in clinical pastoral education. Although this type of supervision is akin to organizational and administrative supervision, it is not one and the same.

Supervision within the hospital organization refers to functions of responsibility for performance and competencies within the organization and the department. The focus of this supervision is not learning. The person being supervised is assumed to be competent in all of the job-related functions assigned to him or her. Of course, if new skills and competencies are required of the employee, the supervisor may assist the individual in meeting these new expectations at an acceptable level.

As a supervisor of clinical pastoral services, the individual is expected to work collaboratively with chaplains to provide quality services. The spiritual care provided is not necessarily reviewed, in depth, as in earlier training days. Rather, the supervisor is available for consultation where situations become complicated due to the nature and types of services required, for problems the primary pastoral care person is having in the delivery of services, and to keep staff informed.

In addition, the supervisor provides a professional evaluation of primary care chaplains. This evaluation is usually based on the individual's job description and on expectations that the organization has of all employees. Any performance problems are addressed through specific behavioral strategies that bring the primary care chaplain up to a minimum performance level.

Example

Reverend Thompson arrived at the hospital with a Masters of Divinity and certificates indicating that he had completed four units of clinical pastoral education. He was ordained in the United Church of Christ and was in good standing with that denomination. He had worked in a parish church for six years and had experience in hospital visitation during that time. At the hospital, he was placed under the supervision of Reverend Smith. He was assigned primarily to pediatrics. He was expected to make regular care visits and be available for emergencies. During the first year, there were several verbal complaints about Reverend Thompson behaving inappropriately with the children. Nothing major was cited, but it was generally felt that Reverend Thompson unnecessarily excited the children and had them moving around in ways that weren't medically safe.

Staff peer observers felt that Reverend Thompson was trying too hard to be a buddy, and not trying hard enough to be a chaplain. On each occasion when this type of complaint was lodged, the supervisor talked with Reverend Thompson. Together they came to an agreement about what behavior was not acceptable. However, the complaints continued. The supervisor felt compelled to include this issue in the annual performance evaluation. Once the problem was identified on the evaluation, a more formal process was begun to evaluate Reverend Thompson's performance and skills as pertained to ministry in pediatrics.

Organizational supervisory skills are usually gained through experience and training. Advanced training covers supervised practice, theory, and conceptual bases for supervision. For example, a typical supervisory development program developed by Jan Roberts, Training Coordinator at New Hampshire Hospital, includes seven learning modules (Roberts, 2000):

1. Introduction to supervision
2. Communication skills
3. Basic facilitation skills
4. Understanding and valuing differences
5. Performance management part I and II
6. Performance appraisal
7. Creating a positive work environment

At the end of the supervisory training program, an individual would have received thirty-two contact hours of continuing education. The individual taking this supervisory training would have completed a pre- and post-self-assessment form such as those provided in Appendixes P and Q.

Administrative Skills Within the Organization

In many hospital settings, the individual chaplain may be required to be a Jack-(or Jill)-of-all-trades. This is often the case in circumstances where there is only one chaplain, or, when there is a conscious determination to place all chaplains on equal footing. For example, a Catholic chaplain and a Protestant chaplain may work parallel to each other from a structural point of view. In situations involving a director of a pastoral care department, all efforts are usually made to hire an individual who has had administrative, as well as supervisory, training and experience.

Administrative functions include the taking of responsibility for all the services within the department. Important management functions include:

- Establishment of vision and mission statements within department
- Leadership and structural management within the hospital
- Establishment of job descriptions and special performance criteria
- Determination of scope of services provided and criteria for the provision of such services
- Maintenance of policies and procedures
- Goal setting and quality improvement projects and processes
- Maintenance of departmental budget
- Selection and supervision of staff
- Maintenance of program

Leadership Within the Organization

The leadership function is one that many chaplains enjoy as they grow in their own professional development. Although it is predominately a call to provide pastoral care that brings most chaplains into hospital ministry, opportunities for growth and development in leadership and training offer ways to grow in other areas. The leadership function is a natural part of the chaplain's role, given the provision of pastoral services to patients, families, colleagues, and others who come into the hospital. In this sense, chaplains, like all employees, are leaders. However, advanced leadership opportunities within the hospital organization can also be developed depending on the hospital's needs, and the chaplain's interests. The following types of leadership roles are common:

- Departmental and supervisory leadership
- New employee training in orientation to spiritual needs
- New employee training and orientation in grief, loss, and recovery

- Customer service improvement team
- Customer service review committee
- Management committees and meetings
- Clinical reviews
- Behavioral management review committee
- Patient family education improvement team and committee
- Programs for patients, peers, and community
- Facilitation and/or leadership of improvement teams
- Ethics committees
- Partners in wellness—patient, family, and team program
- Leadership functions as member of treatment team

Over a period of time, chaplains begin to discover which of these formal and informal aspects of leadership are essential, and which are optional. The chaplain who enjoys leadership roles will make this interest an opportunity to assess personal competencies and preferences when making leadership choices.

Spiritual Care Leadership

One leadership area that chaplains have no choice about becoming well-trained and skilled in is the area of religious and spiritual care, practices, and processes. No matter what the leadership function, the chaplain is always presumed to be a spiritual leader. As a spiritual care leader, one brings spiritual concerns and other value-based issues to bear on organizational and clinical processes. Often, this is accomplished by the same presence used in caring relationships with patients and their families. Presence, in this case, also refers to the representative function of pastoral leadership. At advanced levels, the spiritual care leader is expected to be able to help peers apply spiritual care premises and values at conceptual as well as practical levels. The ability to work with increasingly complex leadership issues, and do so using the language of the organization or various disciplines, is essential.

Typical spiritual care leadership involvement often occurs at points of

- Conflicting values
- Promotion of patient rights
- Empowerment of employees

- Organizational moments of crisis
- Shifting priorities within the organization
- Grief and loss relating to leaders within the organization
- Valuing and recognizing services and service providers
- Authorizing research programs through participation on institutional review boards

CONSULTATION

Entry-level consultation often occurs when the chaplain is a learner or a newcomer. In this position, the chaplain, ideally, takes responsibility to consult with persons in the field regarding standards of care and practice. These standards relate to clinical, pastoral, and organizational processes.

With interest and experience, the chaplain may begin to develop a reputation for being skilled in specific areas. Once certain skills are recognized, the chaplain is bound to find himself or herself being asked to:

- Give as well as receive consults
- Work at the peer level when engaging in a consult
- Consult regarding concerns of other disciplines
- Consult both within and outside the hospital setting on behalf of the hospital
- Consult on issues important to the wider community

An experienced and trained consultant will be skilled in the content of given issues, and the processes integral to those issues. The nature of such a consult would be to:

- Expand knowledge and thinking
- Advise as to standards of professional practice and/or care
- Further processes
- Further resolution and/or planning
- Bring an experienced viewpoint

Consultation, as a service, usually means entering a group or process from a somewhat objective point of view. The consultant is a person with identified skills, who is asked to bring those skills to bear on a certain process within a specified group. Once the consult is finished, the individual leaves the group and discontinues consultant services until requested at another time.

Example

Polly was asked to be a consultant to a group that was having difficulty managing conflict. She was a pastoral counselor and a chaplain, and had much experience managing conflict through the use of systems analysis. Polly arranged to meet with the group's leadership to develop a plan for identifying the conflict, and for helping the group identify processes they could use to work toward resolution.

A year later, the group's leadership called to say that their plan and processes had broken down. They asked if Polly could help once again. She agreed to meet with them a second time, and also agreed to meet with the group. As it turned out, the group had made some headway, but was grieving the changes that had occurred. Polly was able to help the group identify both their accomplishments and their feelings of loss. The group, with Polly's help, devised another plan, and thus this second consultation was also completed. Six months later, the group leaders sent a note to Polly to tell her how much help the consultation had been and to inform her of the group's activities and health.

BIOMEDICAL AND PROFESSIONAL ETHICS

Today, most hospitals have ethics committees, and most chaplains belong to an organization that has a code of professional ethics. In addition, some faith groups also have codes of ethics for their ordained leadership. At minimum, chaplains are expected to know and follow the appropriate code of ethics applying to them. In addition to these personal and professional ethical commitments, some chaplains choose to also become members of the ethics committee within their hospital organization.

In some circumstances, a chaplain needs to become more advanced in the knowledge and practice of professional ethical decision making. This would be the case if:

- The chaplain were to take on leadership functions of an ethics committee
- The chaplain were able to interpret the various codes of ethics for staff, students, or as a consultant
- The chaplain choses to become an expert in this area

ADVANCED PASTORAL CARE

Advanced pastoral care entails specializing in some of the areas noted under brief counseling (see Chapter 1 and Appendix O). Commonly, the pastoral care specialist can specialize in working with age-specific populations such as:

- Children
- Youth
- Adults
- Elders

Chaplains specializing in pastoral care organize their specialization around treatment programs such as:

- Pediatrics
- Oncology
- Psychiatry
- Medical surgical
- Maternity
- Cardiac care
- Substance abuse
- Orthopedics

Chaplains may also choose to specialize in areas of spiritual care. The following areas of spiritual care specialization might be considered:

- Advanced use of pastoral care practices
- Spiritual direction
- Meditation
- Uses of different types of prayers
- World religions and faith traditions
- Spiritual care using holy and sacred scriptures/writings
- Advanced interventions for spiritual distress

The differentiating feature regarding advanced spiritual care is the emphasis put on the ability to get into common care situations and work with greater intensity and focus due to greater knowledge in a chosen area.

ADVANCED PASTORAL COUNSELING

Pastoral counseling at the advanced level is reserved in this book for those who are academically and clinically privileged to provide counseling as a specific modality. Advanced training would need to have occurred in counseling and/or pastoral psychotherapy. In this sense, one refers to the pastoral counselor as one might refer to the clinical psychologist or psychiatric social worker.

Pastoral counseling may include brief counseling, as mentioned in Chapter 7, and may also be seen as a specific type of advanced pastoral care. However, pastoral counseling as a care modality always consists of conducting diagnostic assessments, developing specific treatment plans with specific interventions, and determining ways to evaluate treatment toward the goal of discharge from treatment.

In the hospital setting, there are times when only assessment and diagnosis can occur. In these cases, assumptions can be made that further treatment may happen in an outpatient setting. In some cases, one is able to assess, diagnose, and begin the work of helping the patient become aware of a clinical and/or spiritual problem. In hospitals where patients may stay for several months or even longer, it may be possible to complete sufficient pastoral psychotherapy to motivate the person to engage in additional or follow-up therapy in the community.

Competence in advanced pastoral care may come with continuing education, such as additional units of clinical pastoral education. Competence in pastoral counseling and/or pastoral psychotherapy happens as the result of an additional graduate degree; a specified type of clinical pastoral counseling training (usually by adding at least 1,375 clinical counseling hours), and attainment of certification or licensed levels of professional accomplishment.

Holistic counseling refers to efforts that focus on the interconnection of mind, body, and spirit. Since pastoral counseling focuses on health and healing through the interconnections of all aspects of the person, it is considered holistic. However, in hospitals, standard therapeutic protocols occur even in holistic endeavors. These standards of treatment require prioritization that begins with safety and stabilization of illness, and moves toward wider recovery and health interventions. Figure 8.1 illustrates the progression of care and services from the most focused to the broadest integrative connections.

It is typical for pastoral counseling in the hospital setting to include counseling in the following major areas. In each area, it is assumed that the chaplain would develop an expertise within the area in order to deliver high-quality counseling services.

- Grief, loss, and recovery
- Lifestyle choices
- Relational difficulties
- Spirituality, beliefs, and recovery
- Trauma and recovery
- Wellness through mind, body, and spirit connections

Counseling for Grief, Loss, and Recovery

Grief is a natural response to the loss of a significant person, object, thing, or ideal. Most people recover from grief and loss without any specialized interventions, although the process can take weeks or years to be fully completed. However, complicating factors, feelings, and experiences can make it worthwhile for an individual to receive brief and/or in-depth counseling. Since grief and loss affect the whole person, it is very important for treatment interventions to be holistic.

Mind, body, and spirit healthy connections
Growth, development, and integration
Uncovering and insightful
Practical and solution focused
Coping and symptom management
Safety and stabilization

FIGURE 8.1. Holistic Counseling Priorities

Typical Losses Encountered in Hospital Settings

Most persons entering the hospital come with some sort of loss or anticipation of loss. Except in cases of delivery of an expected and wanted child, most other reasons for hospitalization involve some dysfunction of the body, and people have natural feelings regarding loss of optimum health, no matter how fleetingly.

In a hospital setting losses that tend to benefit from counseling interventions are:

- End of life issues
- Radical changes in life
- Multiple losses
- Possible loss of a child
- Facing illnesses that are accompanied with a social stigma
- Remembrances of complicated issues regarding previous losses
- Impending losses faced alone
- Impending losses that will lead to multiple new losses
- Losses with attached moral issues
- Losses that may cause feelings of significant guilt and shame
- Losses at a time of unstabilized major depression or other major mental or physical illness
- Losses of freedom and choice
- Losses of contact and positive support from families and others

Typical Problems That May Indicate a Need for Counseling

It is not the nature of a particular loss that makes counseling the treatment of choice. Rather, it is the manner in which the individual is managing the resulting grief. Signs that a person, or family, is having difficulty managing grief may include some of the following symptoms or behaviors:

- Absence of feelings or affect for more than several days
- Failure to acknowledge major loss (death, job, need for surgery) so that failure indicates significant risk or problems in functioning
- Excessive rage and uncontrollable hostile behavior
- Severe depression and suicidal thoughts and feelings

- Sustained unwillingness to talk even briefly about thoughts and feelings concerning the loss
- Sustained existential despair
- Failure to be able to plan for discharge

Example 1

Rita entered the acute psychiatric facility in a very disoriented and confused state. She had been found in her home with her spouse who had been dead for several days. Rita was unable to accept that her spouse was dead. She appeared to be experiencing a psychotic breakdown. For a number of months, Rita was essentially unable to care for herself. The focus of treatment was on stabilization through the pharmacological control of psychotic symptoms, and on helping Rita care for herself. It was almost a year before Rita began to realize that her spouse had died and had been cremated. Over the course of the following six months, Rita met with the chaplain who helped her work through her grief to the point at which she could decide what to do with her husband's ashes. Over time, Rita was able to provide better self-care and become reality oriented with some limitations as to her cognitive functioning. She was then discharged.

The chaplain chose to meet twice weekly with Rita. In the beginning, the time spent with her could have been considered pastoral care and support. Over time, the pastoral care work moved into grief counseling. Had Rita been more reality oriented and more talkative, it might have made sense for her to be referred to a loss and recovery group. As it was, she required a one-to-one situation.

Example 2

Bruce was referred to the admissions group for loss and recovery. This group was co-led by the two hospital chaplains who were also pastoral counselors and certified members of the American Association of Pastoral Counselors. One of the two counselors was licensed by the state of New Hampshire.

The referral form from the admissions team came with a diagnosis of an axis one post-traumatic stress disorder. Bruce had many experiences of trauma, and currently was engaged in self-harming behavior.

He was going through a divorce and there were issues of custody of his two children. He refused to accept the divorce and was quite sullen and angry. Additional risk factors identified were substance abuse and suicidal ideation.

Group Therapy Process and Interventions
for Grief and Loss

Group therapy is a common mode of treatment in general and specialized hospitals where enough personnel are available to accept referrals for such treatment. Often, groups conducted in the general hospital setting include outpatients. In an acute inpatient unit, the referrals come from a treatment team. The team, or its designated member, meets with the patient and determines which group or groups might be helpful. The referral is based on diagnosis and problem assessment, and includes documentation of known risk factors that would be helpful to the group leaders (see Appendix R for sample form). Patients are informed that they have been referred to a group.

It is typical for loss and recovery groups to include:

- Introductions of leadership
- Introductions of first names
- Review stages of grief and loss (if new group members are present)
- Opportunities for patients to identify losses
- Opportunities for patients to express thoughts and feelings
- Opportunities for patients to identify where they feel they are in the grieving process

Additional sessions include:

- Assessment and recognition of places where person feels stuck
- Group help for problem areas
- Strategies for coping during early grieving stages
- Strategies for reorganizing life
- Help planning further recovery needs involved in process of discharge and after discharge.
- Role chronic illness may play or has played in loss
- Quality of life and life choices

Recovery Complications

The stages of grief and loss that are used in group processes at New Hampshire Hospital include:

- Shock
- Denial
- Feelings
- Depression
- Reorganization
- Recovery

For more information, the reader is encouraged to read *Grief Education for Caregivers of the Elderly,* particularly Chapter 3, "Bereavement and the Elderly" (McCall, 1999, pp. 41-58). The basic stages and processes that are noted previously and covered in this book can be used for adults of any age.

The phases of loss and recovery are always painful. However, extensive experience in hospital ministry has shown that some processes and situations, are particularly challenging. This is often so in the following circumstances:

- Persons with multiple life challenges have difficulty completing the grief process successfully.
- Persons who have difficulty managing and/or expressing feelings tend to be stuck at that level.
- Persons with a pervasive, depressed stance toward life may have difficulties completely recovering from significant loss. They tend to take all losses equally personally. This applies to persons without clinical depression.
- The decision to "get on with life" happens as a result of successful sorting during the sadness and sorrow of the depression stage. It is often difficult to identify the factors involved in that internal decision to "go on." However, persons who believe in God or a Higher Power, or find some other meaning in life, are likely to be able to make this transition more successfully than those who don't have such beliefs as anchors to life's challenges.
- The stage known as "reorganization" is difficult for most persons. This stage requires new skills, and often people need a

group to act as a coach as they try to acquire the skills needed to reorganize after significant loss.

- It is sometimes difficult to meet the needs of persons who are in the early stages of loss and grief, i.e., shock, denial, feelings and depression, and the needs of members of the group who are in the reorganization and recovery phases. Be that as it may, it is more helpful for the group to have diversity so that individuals have exposure to the process as a whole.

Counseling for Lifestyle Choices

Counseling for lifestyle choices is another area where pastoral counseling resources can be helpful in the hospital setting. A frequent result of hospitalization is the need to make significant changes upon returning home. Change itself is difficult to accomplish, even when it is sought. However, changes that must be made in a reactive manner—as a response to a problem—seem to be even more difficult. In addition to the grief and loss response, there is the added complication of the motivation, insight, and practice required when learning something new, even if it is good for you.

Example

Eunice entered the hospital weighing three times what would be considered a normal, healthy weight. In addition to a weight problem, she had symptoms of moderate depression and a history of psychosis. She felt unloved and unlovable. One focus of treatment was her weight. She was put on a restricted calorie program, and consequently, was frequently hungry as well as depressed. She was unclear about how people really felt about her, let alone how she felt about herself. She believed in God and felt God was with her but was punishing her in some way. She certainly considered dieting a punishment, even though the medical staff tried to convince her that it was medically necessary, as her weight was a threat to her health and well-being. Everything became just one more loss to her.

Eunice was referred to the loss and recovery group where she found a supportive atmosphere, leadership who understood the processes of grief and loss, and found a therapeutic model for helping individuals make significant changes in their lives.

In addition to understanding the stages and processes of grief and loss, the group leaders also referred to a model of change developed by James Prochaska, John Norcross, and Carlo DiClemente, in *Changing for Good* (1994, p. 39). They describe six stages of change:

1. Precontemplation
2. Contemplation
3. Preparation
4. Action
5. Maintenance
6. Termination

This model for change was helpful to Eunice, and works quite well with loss and recovery issues. It also works for individuals facing the need to make a variety of changes.

Typical Problematic Areas Requiring Lifestyle Changes

- Nutrition and exercise changes
- Stress reduction
- Developing spiritual care practices
- Problematic relationships
- Response to chronic illness management
- Repetitive self-defeating behaviors
- Establishing a more balanced lifestyle
- Use of spiritual resources to change addictive behavior

Relational Difficulties

Relational difficulties might also be a focus for pastoral counseling while a person is in a hospital setting. When counseling is indicated, the pastoral counselor is likely to use systems theory, a form of behavioral therapy, and perhaps the Self-in-Relation Model developed at the Stone Center in Wellesley, Massachusetts. Interventions involving relationship issues are most likely to occur on a one-to-one basis or in the context of family. Groups that deal with coping skills, support for specified illnesses, grief, loss, and recovery, are also contexts for working with relational issues.

Example

Cherie came to the hospital with a "bout" of depression. She was confined to a psychiatric ward for some time, and tried to relax and make the best of it. It was difficult. She found that she was often severely depressed, even suicidal. When that was not the case, she was angry with her husband whom she felt did not understand or support her. In fact, he had said that she had better get her act together, and soon, or he was walking out the door. Cherie was not overly religious, but she did believe in God and felt challenged in her faith, her family, and her health. She was referred to a chaplain/pastoral counselor.

Typical Problematic Relational Areas

- Family cut-offs or disconnections
- Family enmeshments or lack of role definition and room for individuality
- Abuse and/or neglect within the family—past or present
- Deficits in capacity or skill
- Burnout of caregiving members of the family
- Over or underfunctioning by various members
- Emotional unavailability
- Broken marriage or broken partnership vows/agreements
- Lack of understanding and acceptance of illness and health issues
- Responses to major/chronic illnesses
- Conflict within the relationship
- Conflicting beliefs and faith systems

Counseling Concerning Spirituality, Beliefs, and Recovery

A crisis of meaning, purpose, and direction is commonplace when a person is faced with a challenging illness. When the physical brain and body are struggling for balance, it makes sense that some form of spiritual distress will occur. The chaplain with pastoral counseling training skills is uniquely qualified to take on complicated spiritual issues in the context of counseling. Complicated spiritual issues are usually discovered through an in-depth assessment of an individual's life experiences and beliefs surrounding the illness and the challenges he or she is facing.

Example 1: A Vengeful God

A bright, attractive, young woman sat in the loss and recovery group with her legs stretched out and her eyes bright and attentive. As the stages of loss and grief were identified, she insisted that the stage we now refer to as "emotions" was really "anger," and she said that she had trouble with feeling anger. She described numerous losses and tragedies in her young life, and stated, amidst rage and tears, that her anger was with God for allowing all these things to happen to her. She declared emphatically that she hated God, that "he was mean and vicious." She went on to say that God was like the door on the therapy room, "God is no more to me than a wooden door that throws thunderbolts."

It would not have helped to defend God. Besides, that's not really the pastoral role. In fact, it was the young woman who needed protection. She just didn't know that she needed protection—from people, from the harsh realities of human limitations, and from not being able to absolutely control her destiny. I encouraged her to express her feelings directly to God while sitting in this group of supportive women. She tried, but could only speak about God (He does this, etc.). She could not speak to God (I hate you). It was a step, however, for her to say what she did in the circle of people and chaplain.

Example 2: An Abandoning God

Marie sat in the conversations with the chaplains group and rubbed her forehead. She said she was feeling very sick that day. She was still losing weight, and was not permitted to stay in her room. "If I had my way," she said, "I'd stay in my room all day and never come out. That's why I'm here." When asked by another member of the group about what church she went to, she declared with great conviction, "When they took away my child I knew that there was no God."

Example 3: The Dark Night of the Soul

The family gathered in the intensive care waiting area feeling helpless and alone. They waited to hear whether Cecil would survive the heart attack. It was a Catholic hospital, but they certainly weren't Catholic. Years ago, Cecil's wife and daughter had attended the Assembly of God church in the little town where they had lived. If anyone had asked them now, they would have said they didn't go to church. They believed in heaven but were no longer sure how that worked. Besides, they were afraid that maybe Cecil didn't qualify for salvation. After all, he never had attended church. In fact, he had been known to scoff at it.

On the third night of hospitalization, Cecil died. Three months later, his daughter Catherine was hospitalized for severe depression. She had trouble sleeping and eating, and had continuing nightmares about falling into the flames of hell. She couldn't shake the sense of impending doom and her feelings of unworthiness. She had no previous episodes of depression and was given an antidepressant that had not worked as well as they had hoped. She was referred for pastoral counseling.

Beliefs That May Complicate Recovery

- Conflicting belief systems
- Lack of awareness of a belief in anything
- Existential despair
- Inability to experience hope
- Guilt and shame
- Making health care decisions against one's beliefs
- Psychotic intrusion of religious material that leads to grandiosity or unsafe practices
- Change in ability to engage in spiritual practices with satisfaction, meaning, or pleasure
- Feelings that God has abandoned them
- Feelings of being singled out for punishment or to be taught a lesson
- Beliefs that one has to do everything oneself

Counseling for Trauma and Recovery

Persons may be hospitalized with histories of sexual abuse, physical abuse, and neglect. They may have experienced rape or other violent acts. They may have observed such violence. These intrusive, violent experiences may become major causes of illness, and they may also be factors in a person's difficulties in recovering from illnesses.

The recovery from trauma involves a significant healing that must include spiritual work along with relational and emotional work. Behavioral, expressive, psychodynamic, and pastoral counseling are all modalities that can be used in this kind of work. Often individuals are assessed for trauma and receive some psychoeducation and brief stabilization counseling in the hospital setting. In cases of a short hospitalization, the patient will be referred for further help. Sometimes, a person who has a complicated trauma history may remain in a psychiatric unit for a period of several months to a year. In these cases, more intense counseling occurs in individual and group therapy programs.

Example

Robin was hospitalized because of a suicide attempt. She was diagnosed with post-traumatic stress disorder, and it was possible that a personality disorder made stable relationships difficult. She felt that she had a problem controlling her feelings, but she wasn't quite sure about the mood disorder. In group therapy, she talked about a relationship that she felt had crossed professional boundaries. She was extremely angry and fearful. She was also ambivalent about her positive feelings toward the person. The group was able to affirm that she had sought help and told her that was a good first step. The leader helped Robin calm down by using a deep breathing technique during a particularly difficult part of the session. It was clear to everyone, including Robin, that further counseling would be important.

Counseling for Wellness Through Mind, Body, and Spirit Connections

Often, group and individual counseling in the hospital setting focuses on gaining or regaining balance, harmony, and/or wellness. A particularly successful inpatient group program might involve guest co-leaders from different disciplines. A nutritionist, an expressive art therapist, a spiritual care professional, and a physical therapist are examples of professionals who might be brought into such therapeutic endeavors. Persons who are struggling in the spiritual care portion of wellness can be referred for individual counseling as appropriate. It is crucial in this work to be practical, to identify obstacles, and be resources for spiritual recovery.

Example

Dave was not sure he wanted to attend the wellness group that was held in the gym. He really didn't care if he got well or not, especially if it meant making changes in his lifestyle. He certainly wasn't going to give up smoking, or eating pizza and donuts. He never could stand exercise anyway. Besides, the Bible never said that he would live forever. He went to the group because he thought it was easier than dealing with the flack he would receive if he did not go. When the co-leader was introduced, he was surprised to find that it was the chaplain. He had never heard of spiritual care and spiritual practices, so he found himself listening. He had some reservations though. He wondered about how his beliefs fit in with nutrition and exercise, but he was embarrassed to bring it up in the group. He did mention his reservations to the leader privately, and was referred for pastoral counseling.

Typical Mind, Body, and Spirit Disconnections

- Believing that faith has nothing to do with health care
- Making spiritual care decisions that one is trying to keep secret and really don't seem to fit in with one's faith group
- Thinking that it's all a matter of mind over body or spirit

TRAINING PROGRAMS, TEACHING, AND SUPERVISION

Another area for specialization in the hospital ministry field is that of educator and supervisor. Normally, clinical pastoral educators in the hospital setting belong to clinical pastoral care organizations and/or clinical pastoral counseling organizations. The programs run by these educators may include the training of seminarians, lay ministers, and other persons specializing in advanced pastoral care or counseling. Many hospital organizations believe that they benefit from such programs. Certainly, chaplains who choose to specialize in the training of other spiritual care and counseling providers, feel that training and supervision adds to their desire to keep fresh and up to date in the field. It also helps to provide a career ladder within the field and within the hospital organization.

CONTRIBUTIONS TO THE FIELD—
RESEARCH AND WRITING

It is less common for chaplains and pastoral counselors in the hospital setting to engage in research and writing. However, this type of practice is needed. Certainly, it is easier to develop research and writing skills in a research or teaching hospital. In these settings, one can often collaborate with professionals from other disciplines on joint projects, and in so doing, support and mentor one another.

If you are interested in engaging in research or writing in the health care field, you may wish to consider these suggestions:

- Find out who is conducting research at your hospital
- Find out who has published at your hospital
- Talk with persons who have published and are members of your professional organization
- Make a list of areas that you have learned something about
- List areas in which you excel
- List areas in which resources are lacking
- Find a friend with whom to share your dream
- Start gathering data
- Start writing

INTERPRETATION AND ADVOCACY
WITHIN THE WIDER COMMUNITY

As a result of the wide variety of skills developed within the hospital ministry profession, one often finds opportunities to bring some of these skills to the larger community. An individual who has specialized in interpretation and advocacy of mind, body, and spirit in the health care field will sometimes bring this focus and its surrounding values and beliefs to bear at worship, in church settings, and in educational efforts within other disciplines.

DEVELOPING A PROFESSIONAL PLAN
FOR GROWTH AND DEVELOPMENT

In order for a pastoral care chaplain/counselor to continue to thrive professionally, it is important to develop a long-term plan for professional growth. The risk of fatigue, emotional strain, and burnout on the pastoral caregiver's part makes a review of his or her original mission statement and core beliefs essential. Any changes can be noted in the current plan. It is helpful to make an assessment of where one is in ministry, and where one wishes to be in the next several years.

In developing this plan, one might ask some of the following questions:

1. What do I like and dislike about my job?
2. What would I like to learn to do better?
3. If I were to move to a different pastoral care job, what area would I choose?
4. Do I want to do what I am doing now for the next five years?
5. How much risk in time, money, and effort am I willing to undertake in order to make changes that involve training or certification?
6. What kind of education and skills would help me do what I want to do better?

Chapter 9

Making Connections

A rebuilding of the relationship between human services and the church at both the local and the system level could lead to improved outcomes—psychosocial and spiritual. The balm in Gilead, the soothing of one's soul, is best experienced as an inner sense of peace and hope nurtured and strengthened by a supportive community. (Bussema and Bussema, 2000, pp. 123-124)

One of the most striking aspects of hospital ministry is the teamwork involved; one quickly learns that everyone is a member of a team. One also learns that each team is somehow connected to other teams that must all work together to promote health and well-being. It takes time and commitment to make sure that these connections happen. It also takes time to discern which connections will be most beneficial in any given situation.

Health and healing are the results of a mind, body, and spiritual connectedness that promotes harmony through peaceful and effective life functioning. Disconnection at personal, interpersonal, and communal levels leads to imbalance and stress, and may sometimes lead to disease. To combat disease, it is vitally important that we understand that all of life has a rhythm and interconnectedness. These interconnections, while often strong for many people, can be quite fragile and easily broken. Therefore, it is no surprise to find that positive and healthy interconnectedness is essential for all living persons.

THE LARGE PICTURE OF SERVICE

Service, in hospital ministry, is based on a commitment to help patients, organizations, systems, and communities become connected through efforts that promote health and healing for all. This commitment to making practical connections has been an underlying goal of this practical guide to hospital ministry. Too often we focus on illness or problems such as cancer, abortion, depression, and heart surgery, and we miss the larger context of what true connectedness means to processes of health and healing. For true connectedness to happen, we need to understand that persons, organizations, and systems are all crucial components in the central task of creating healthy mind, body, and spirit-filled living.

Persons engaged in hospital ministry are usually quite used to focusing on connections and disconnections in a person's health or lack of health. In any given situation, it is common for a chaplain or spiritual care provider to identify possible connections that could be helpful to an individual in the process of his or her recovery. Other connective possibilities, such as legal, insurance/financial coverage, and research and development efforts might also be considered. The following list, however, contains basic essential connections to be considered when helping people recover.

Making Healthy and Healing Connections

- Through a global mind, body, and spirit of health care and healing
- Through state and national health care teams and processes
- Through community organizational health care teams
- Through the church and/or faith community
- Through community clergy, lay, and spiritual caregivers
- Through hospital organizational teams
- Through hospital patient care and treatment teams
- Through pastoral care teams
- Through chaplains and spiritual care providers
- Through family and friends
- Through self of patient/healer
- Through personal and transpersonal mind, body, and spirit of health and healing

Example

Arlene entered the hospital with severe depression and had not been taking care of herself. She was not eating and was hearing voices that berated her. She believed these voices came from Satan. Her torment was great. She belonged to a church and normally attended weekly worship. This particular church had some guidelines about living that included preferences concerning which foods to eat and not to eat. While in the hospital, Arlene agonized over taking medication and the lack of a healthy lifestyle that she believed was crucial to Christian living. She had never had a psychiatric illness and was unprepared for a lengthy recovery process.

During the course of hospitalization, Arlene worked closely with the chaplain, who with Arlene's permission, contacted her clergyperson to inquire about that church's stance on taking medication and other health-related issues. This information was given to Arlene and the treatment team. At first, the treatment team thought that some of the lifestyle issues (such as fresh air, daily walks, and a largely vegetarian diet) were just examples of Arlene's refusal to cooperate and part of her neurotic guilt pattern. For example, they particularly noted that she ate pork, even though she felt intensely guilty about it. After listening to the kind of healthy lifestyle that Arlene's church recommended, and realizing that some of these things actually related to spiritual care understandings held by the church as a whole, the team came to a better understanding of what holistic healing might mean for her.

The team endeavored to help Arlene manage her psychotic and depressive symptoms, while helping her find ways to integrate spiritual care practices that made sense to her. When she was released from the hospital, persons in the community were brought in, and assisted in helping Arlene keep up these positive spiritual care practices at home. For some time she continued to receive mental health care that included integration of spiritual care practices. Arlene truly needed to have health care professionals, friends, and her church understand and help her in a healing process that respected and integrated what was important to her.

HOSPITAL-WIDE SPIRITUAL CARE EFFORTS

Previous chapters have focused on the central role of the patient and the various roles and functions of chaplains and other spiritual care providers in hospital ministry. However, spiritual care, in its broadest definition, is not the sole task or domain of the chaplain or professional spiritual care provider. Others also provide spiritual care directly or indirectly. From this perspective, care that integrates spiritual beliefs and practices can hopefully be found in various hospital functions and activities.

Example

One afternoon about twenty-five employees gathered in a conference room to say good-bye to a member of the medical staff. Everyone asked where the doctor was going and what his plans were for the future. A wonderful cake was cut, and those who wished to say something were invited to do so. Several persons spoke kindly of the doctor and one or two told a humorous story of times gone by. Finally, a gift was opened and the medical director spoke. The medical director spoke of the doctor's work and of his commitment to working on behalf of those who needed care and advocacy. He paraphrased one of Jesus' statements about "the kingdom" being within each of us and suggested that this departing doctor certainly seemed to be able to look for that "kingdom" in the individuals he served as well as the organizations and systems he sought to change.

A Chaplain's Duty

While persons from other disciplines may choose to integrate some aspect of spiritual care, beliefs, and values into their functioning, the chaplain is expected to do so. In this sense, the chaplain is always on duty. There are many events and processes within the organization that typically involve chaplains. Patient care and the spiritual care provided to families and significant others is of course the chaplain's primary task.

Other duties and expectations arise within the hospital as an organization. These duties promote healthy and welcomed supportive connections with other employees within the hospital, and provide a ministry to the organization. Typical times when a chaplain is likely to be called to minister to and with staff include:

- Hospital functions: Invocations and/or prayers
- Critical care moments with staff
- Critical care moments with related organizations
- Memorial services for staff/employees

- Occasional weddings and baptisms for staff/employees
- Ethics committee

Other Opportunities for Involvement

In the larger context of the hospital as organizational system, chaplains may find themselves involved in numerous ways. Some of this involvement may or may not appear, at first glance, to be a direct responsibility of chaplains. At times, the chaplain will volunteer based on personal and professional needs and interests. At other times the chaplain is identified within the organization as having the skills needed. Some of the various types of additional involvement within the hospital system include:

- Wellness efforts for staff, families, and patients
- Patient-family education and support services
- Manager's meetings
- Physician support groups
- Customer service committees/teams
- Behavioral management review committees
- Library committees and reviews

COMMUNITY CLERGY INVOLVEMENT

All hospitals are used to having clergy visit with patients. However, each hospital is unique in approaches to pastoral care from outside sources. The differences range from treating clergy as one would treat any other visitor, to considering community clergy as professional colleagues. These differences can be somewhat confusing and often frustrating to clergy who have been trained to consider themselves as privileged by virtue of their ordained status.

Community clergy and spiritual care providers may visit patients under several circumstances. The primary reason is usually because the patient is a member of one's faith group. Second, area clergy may visit patients at the request of family members and friends. Third, clergy are often called upon to visit patients who are of the same faith tradition but without a local pastor, rabbi, or priest. When clergy are asked by the hospital to make such visits, they act as informal (usually unpaid) consultants. Clergy may also choose to volunteer their services. When clergy act as volunteers, they are under the responsibility and supervision of the hospital's pastoral care department.

Because many clergy have had one or more units of clinical pastoral education, they often expect the same role and response when they come to the hospital as community clergy. However, they are not in the same situation. As students they were temporarily part of the hospital team and had access to patients in the role of student-chaplains. They were under the supervision of a staff chaplain and had to abide by hospital processes and procedures. These student chaplains had relatively easy access to other employees, to the patients' charts, and to participation in patient care/treatment reviews. These students, as all hospital employees, were bound by rules of confidentiality regarding information about patients.

When clergy from the community come to the hospital, their access to information about patients is usually limited to what the patient, or patient's family, wishes to disclose. Under normal circumstances, hospital personnel are not able to release any information without the patient's written consent. This does not mean that hospital personnel are unwilling to relate to community clergy, nor does it mean that the health care team is unappreciative of having clergy provide pastoral care to patients and their families. Most ward staff are delighted to have a person's pastor, priest, or rabbi present in a supportive role.

Suggestions for Community Clergy and Pastoral Caregivers

- Get to know your community hospital and any hospital that you are likely to visit to provide pastoral care. Ask for a tour.
- Get to know the chaplains and spiritual care providers who are on staff and get to know departmental procedures. Ask for an orientation to pastoral care and for some formal or informal training about specific policies and procedures that the department and the hospital might have, and how these procedures might apply to you when you visit patients at the hospital.
- Attend open houses and in-services that the hospital or pastoral care departments may offer.
- Let pastoral care departments, staff chaplains know what voluntary services you might be able to provide. In hospitals with no

staff chaplains, give this information to the hospital administration.

- If you feel that you have not been treated hospitably during your pastoral care visit, consult with the staff chaplain or the department of pastoral care. Often this type of consultation can help you on future visits. If no chaplaincy services exist, ask to speak with someone from administration or the director of patient care.
- When you enter the hospital, wear an identification badge of some sort, and be prepared to be flexible should the patient that you are visiting be unavailable or unwilling to have you visit.
- Once you are engaged in a hospital visit, it is expected that you will follow professional procedures such as are suggested in Chapter 7, which considers basic skill development for chaplains. If you are not acquainted with these processes and skills, it may be a good idea to consider further education.

Suggested Procedures for Community Clergy

Hospitals often rely heavily on community clergy involvement in their pastoral care program. To encourage clergy and promote partnership, it is helpful to have a specific protocol in place for these professionals. An example of such a protocol follows:

New Clergy Protocol for Hospital Visitation

1. New clergy contacts hospital chaplain to set up appointment for orientation (Chaplain may also initiate meeting)
2. At hospital orientation:
   - Conversation with chaplain regarding previous ministry/clinical pastoral education experience
   - Description of facilities and resources at hospital
   - Tour of hospital with emphasis on locations visiting clergy may visit—emergency department, cardiac care unit, oncology, medical/surgical, pre-op holding room
   - introductions to staff and any unique protocols such as length of cardiac care unit visits, phone from waiting room first policies, etc.

- View video on confidentiality; read hospital policy on "Statement of Responsibility/Confidentiality," and sign last page (Same as all hospital employees and interns)
- Interview with hospital employee health department for tuberculosis test, and immunization check (Same as volunteers and interns)
- Receive cardboard "Visiting Clergy" sign or sticker with hospital logo to place on dashboard of car while using clergy parking space
- Go to human resources to have picture taken for visiting clergy badge, fill out form

3. The name of the clergy and congregation will be placed on the pastoral care call list, if it is not already there. Now, this congregation can be called by pastoral care volunteers to notify them of members who are in the hospital and have identified themselves as part of this congregation.

4. Having received this orientation and signed the statement of responsibility/confidentiality includes this clergy in the hospital loop of privileged communication. It does not allow the clergy to write a note in the chart or read the patient record. It does, however, allow the hospital staff to respond to questions the clergy may have regarding the patient's condition, prognosis, and status with family. The rapport that builds with staff over the years also increases the availability of information regarding the patient's condition.

THE USE OF CLERGY CONSULTANTS

Every hospital relies on clergy consultants to some degree. Clergy are considered consultants for the purposes of hospital ministry when they are asked to provide pastoral care services to persons who are not part of their congregation. These consultants often represent faith traditions not represented by staff chaplains. In some cases, the hospital has no chaplains, and relies solely on consultants and clergy who have parishioners in the hospital. Consultants can be formally organized within a pastoral care department, or they can be informally called upon as needed. Consultants can be paid a fee for service, or they can provide consultative services as part of their church, denomination, faith traditions, or personal expectations and wishes.

While it may not be possible to quote research concerning the factors that cause clergy to serve as consultants, some possible factors include the following.

Factors in Community Clergy's Decisions to Be Consultants in a General Hospital

- Support of a person from one's faith tradition, even though he or she is not a member of one's church
- Previous clinical pastoral training and interest
- Viewed as part of clergy ministry to community
- Perceived closeness to hospital chaplains
- Interest in working with persons who have specific diseases
- Time available for at-large hospital ministry
- Support of congregation for this type of ministry
- Expectations of faith tradition
- Confidence and comfort in providing consultative services
- Amount of demand placed on person as consultant
- Being paid versus volunteering

Factors in Community Clergy's Decisions to Be Consultants in a Psychiatric Hospital

- Previous clinical pastoral training in psychiatric setting and interest
- Viewed as part of clergy ministry to community
- Perceived closeness to hospital chaplains
- Interest in working with persons who have mental illness
- Time available for at-large hospital ministry
- Support of congregation for this type of ministry
- Expectations of faith tradition
- Confidence and comfort in providing consultative services
- Amount of demand placed on person as consultant
- Being paid versus volunteering

Factors That May Hinder Community Clergy's Decisions
to Be Consultants in a Psychiatric Hospital

- Lack of knowledge about mental illness
- The prevalent stigma attached to mental illness and psychiatric hospitals
- The strict confidential policies adhered to by psychiatric facilities
- The estrangement psychiatric patients may have from churches
- The possible unpredictability of the patient during pastoral care visits

Steps for Setting Up a System of Having Community Clergy
and Spiritual Care Providers As Consultants

1. Decide if you need a formal or informal consulting system.
2. Determine what service could or would be desired from a consultant.
3. Determine if funds are available to pay consultants for their services or if this will be a voluntary effort.
4. Determine how consultants will fit into the structure of the pastoral care department. Who will be their contact person? Who will supervise their work?
5. Determine what kind of training is needed for consultants and any other policies and procedures that might be involved. How will referrals be made? Will the person sign a confidentiality form? Is an orientation required? How will feedback happen?
6. Determine a process for selecting consultants and negotiating formal or informal agreements.

CHURCH AND FAITH COMMUNITY
BRIDGE BUILDING

According to Margaret Kornfeld, a pastoral counselor and current president of the American Association of Pastoral Counselors,

> Authentic community is the "medicine" our society needs. We and other mental health professionals know that loneliness, isolation, emptiness, and a sense of meaninglessness are the frequent

complaints of those coming for help. . . . We know that people can find healing in community because we have witnessed such healing. . . . We have seen them come alive. We have watched them make close friendships in the community in which they experienced their wholeness. (Kornfeld, 1998, pp. 16-17)

Health, healing, and wholeness take place in the midst of circles of community. The hospital setting is but one circle of the health care community. Family and close friends forms another circle of community. Other circles of community are found within the contexts of jobs, volunteer opportunities, social groupings, political endeavors, and shared interests and hobbies. Wherever one finds healthy and life-giving contacts, one finds circles of community with possibilities for experiencing healing and wholeness.

The church used to be a central circle of community for many people. It still is for some. But times have changed. This change is evidenced in hospital ministry. Now, one is careful when one asks about church, religious affiliations, or even faith traditions. It is not always politically correct to do so in society, or in the health care system. In fact, it is sometimes more politically correct of speak of spirituality, spiritual care and practices, and of any other religion besides the Christian religion, in the health care field. One learns of this dilemma early in one's training.

Example

Nursing students come each semester for their psychiatric rotation at New Hampshire Hospital. Part of the rotation involves a general awareness of therapeutic opportunities for patients. Since pastoral services provides therapeutic opportunities, students frequently ask to sit in during groups. On this particular day, a student nurse asked to sit in on the conversations with the chaplains group.

It happened that two patients believed in God, but had no use for religion. The third patient confessed that she was quite angry with God and had crossed "him" off her list. When the student nurse was asked what she believed, she replied, "I don't think it is important to go to church, but having your own spiritual beliefs can be helpful." After the group, she mentioned to the chaplain leader that she had been uncomfortable responding to the patient. She was a Catholic, but didn't know if she should reveal this or if she should support religion and church attendance.

One also learns to be a bit skeptical about clergy. The biggest fear that some health care professionals have about clergy and volunteers from specific faith groups is that they will force certain beliefs on patients against their wishes. In all fairness, some faith traditions focus on conversion and evangelizing as a preferred way of providing pastoral care. However, it is equally true that a large segment of persons hospitalized in this country still come from Judeo-Christian faith traditions, and many persons come from conservative and evangelical churches. Religious tolerance of these conservative and evangelical traditions is just as essential to health care as diversity and honoring individualized spiritual beliefs and preferences.

Still it is the task of hospitals and of pastoral care chaplains to reach out to the community, churches and faith groups within their communities. It is hospital ministry's responsibility to build part of this partnership bridge for the sake of health and well-being for all persons. The following are bridge-building suggestions from the hospital side of the partnership.

The Hospital Ministry Side of the Bridge

- Upon admissions, hospital chaplains and other designated persons should ask about religious preferences and faith traditions (if any). A careful noting of typical answers should be used to improve choices noted on care forms.
- Patients who note religious preferences should be asked if they would like to have their pastor, priest, rabbi, elder, practitioner, or other faith community leader notified of their hospitalization.
- Patients need to be allowed to express their beliefs, doubts, feelings, and concerns about their faith and faith communities. In many cases, the chaplain will be able to help and encourage the patient to be somehow connected with a preferred faith community.
- Chaplains need to know about various faith traditions so they can be reasonably informed about certain traditions.
- Chaplains need to be respectful of all faith groups. In cases where a person may be interested or involved with cults, a chap-

lain will of course want to help the patient be careful when making choices. It is most helpful in these circumstances to talk about safety and self-care.

• Whenever possible, a chaplain needs to try to help persons connect to churches when they want to do so. Knowing about the people and strengths of specific churches can be very helpful when making referrals.

• Whenever possible, a chaplain refers a person to more than one church.

• Whenever possible, a chaplain teaches patients about getting along in a church community. This teaching includes what to expect, how to handle concerns, how to approach clergy and elders, and how to decide what kind of involvement would be helpful.

The chaplain's part of building a bridge with faith communities also involves reaching out to churches and faith groups. The chaplain may be a guest preacher, a guest speaker, or an educational resource. Some chaplains join interfaith groups that are located in their hospital's region. Basically, a chaplain wants to convey that "we are interested in you" and " we hope you are interested in us."

A partnership requires more than one partner. Thus, it is crucial that the church and other faith traditions reach out to hospitals in their midst. It is crucial that the church help promote health care. The church has a part in the bridge-building business too.

Example

Recently, I received an e-mail from a clergyperson with a request for someone to come to her church during National Pastoral Care Week to speak about mental illness from a personal/professional perspective. She had received materials from her faith group, the United Church of Christ, and was looking forward to having a service using some materials provided. She was aware that there would likely be members of her church who had experiences with mental illness, and others who have had family members and friends with similar experiences. She wanted the homily to be meaningful, and felt that a message that moved people to be involved would be helpful.

The Church's Side of the Bridge to Health Care

- Churches and faith communities need to recover a sense of power that comes from faith and spiritual care practices.
- Many churches have a lay ministry program for parishioners. It would be a good idea to have a hospital ministry program as part of their outreach to those not from one's own parish.
- Churches need to openly discuss and discern their role in promoting health and healing. Many churches have healing services.
- Churches and church members often provide a volunteer resource to hospitals that is invaluable and provides members with opportunities to witness health care.
- Churches need to consider follow-up care for persons hospitalized. It makes sense for churches to have trained individuals work with those recovering from illness. The collaborative development of a spiritual/health care plan makes sense.
- The church can be an appropriate advocate for holistic health care.
- The church can help its leaders and clergy with time for continuing education and with assessment as to pastoral care strengths and limitations.
- The church can designate hospitals that are part of their expected pastoral care coverage of clergy and laypersons.
- The church can support health care providers (nurses, doctors, etc.) who are members of their congregation in working with the chaplain in the hospital.

THE REWARDS OF HOSPITAL MINISTRY

The first time I entered a hospital on behalf of a local congregation, I was thirty-four years old and the year was 1980. I was confidently visiting hospitalized members of my church. I had had no clinical pastoral training but did have much compassion and common sense. I was a good listener and asked what I could do. I tried to be optimistic whenever possible, and tears would fill my eyes when situations were horrendous and life threatening. I was moved by a sense of call and a desire to be connected with people in need of the connections of their faith and their faith community.

In 1982, I took the first of eight units of clinical pastoral education. I visited patients in geriatric centers, general hospital settings, and in a psychiatric hospital. I was amazed by the resiliency and strength of patients, families, and staff in challenging situations. I became aware of the challenges and traumatic events that seemed too much for the human spirit to bear. In the years that followed, I became aware of my own challenges and resiliency. That awareness was a secondary gain to helping patients, families, and staff.

In 1983, I began taking my first pastoral counseling courses and started an extensive program of clinical pastoral counseling training. I learned how to integrate health care theories with practical, focused interventions that often led to changes in coping, and even healing and recovery. I also learned that in some cases, the final stages of healing and recovery needed to be left to the patient and to God. I learned about true hope and the depths of despair and helplessness. Little by little, I was rewarded with growing feelings of competence and increasing faith in the work I was being called to do. I gained colleagues, mentors, and circles of communities that shared my interest in health and healing.

By 1994, I was supervising and training students in pastoral counseling. Some of this training took place in a pastoral counseling center, and some took place in a psychiatric hospital. In becoming an educator and mentor, I was rewarded by being able to teach and learn from students. I began writing and engaging in community teaching and advocacy. I began to feel the effects of my contributions and the contributions of others.

Rewards, as with most meaningful things, are in the eye of the beholder. However, the eye of the beholder changes, as does every living thing. What one chaplain would consider a reward for engaging in hospital ministry might not be a reward for another chaplain. What may be at the top of one's list may be in the middle or at the bottom of another's list.

I've heard colleagues say:

- I am doing this until I learn ministry, then I'll return to the church.
- I am here to work with patients.

- I like supervising students and running a clinical training program.
- I believe God called me to hospital ministry, so here I am.
- I love working in an ecumenical setting.
- The church is just too closed-minded in its thinking; I've found a home here.
- Jesus gave us a mandate to visit and care for the sick. This is my work as a Christian.
- I came and I stayed.

The importance of a discernment of call to hospital ministry is crucial for the individual and for the persons served. It is this discernment of call, and meaning, that leads chaplains and spiritual care providers to grow in skill, development of professional identities, and in the provision of quality services. It can be said that the context of care in hospital ministry is always found in the living matrix of connective circles of quality caring events. This book is just one of those containers that provide a crucible for growth and development and for health and healing!

Appendix A

Categorization of Hospital Ministry Form

Name	Defining Criteria	Training Source	Service Delivered	Compe-tencies	Patients Served

Appendix B

Pastoral Services Spiritual Care and Chaplain Request Form

Name: _____   Date: _____

Unit: _____

You may request one of the following services with a check mark.

_____ Initial visit

_____ Worship information

_____ Pastoral care visit

_____ Counseling

_____ Prayer

_____ Communion

_____ Holy Communion for Catholics

_____ Literature and Bibles

_____ Cross/Rosary

_____ Family support

_____ Spiritual care resources

Please leave this form at the nurse's station on your unit.

Appendix C

What Patients Request
on Chaplain Request Forms

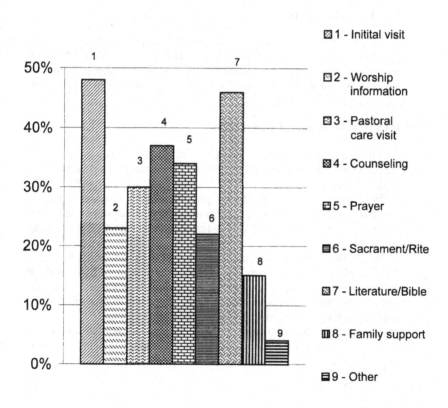

1 - Initital visit

2 - Worship information

3 - Pastoral care visit

4 - Counseling

5 - Prayer

6 - Sacrament/Rite

7 - Literature/Bible

8 - Family support

9 - Other

Appendix D

Sample Pastoral Services
Policy Statement

I. POLICY TITLE: Pastoral Services Policy and Procedures

II. POLICY STATEMENT:

It is the policy of the Pastoral Services Department to serve the spiritual needs of the patients of New Hampshire Hospital through quality pastoral care. This service shall extend to family members, visitors, hospital staff, affiliated on-campus clinical programs, and to the community at large.

III. PASTORAL CARE PHILOSOPHY:

The Pastoral Services Department supports a compassionate and caring approach to patients, family members, visitors, and co-workers at the hospital.

We believe a total patient care plan recognizes that every person has psychosocial, economic, spiritual, and physical needs, and that identifying and meeting these needs contributes to the total well-being of patients.

While the Pastoral Services Department assesses, plans for, provides, and evaluates our services in light of individual, group, and the institution's spiritual needs, we do so within the total hospital care system. Working within this system, we endeavor to provide quality care for elders, adults, young adults, and children.

Members of the Pastoral Services Department shall adhere to the code of ethics of their respective religious affiliations and professional associations.

IV. DEFINITIONS:

A. Spiritual Needs—refers to a person's faith, well-being, feelings, and thoughts as they relate to the person's life functioning. Faith may involve an understanding of God and/or the meaning, purpose, or direction in life.

B. Pastoral Care—refers to clinical interventions by Pastoral Services staff and trainees which invite and motivate healthy and meaningful use of each person's beliefs and attitudes.

C. Pastoral Counseling—refers to a process in which hospital pastoral counselors and trainees utilize insights and principles derived from the disciplines of theology and behavioral sciences to work with persons toward the achievement of wholeness and health.

D. Dangerously Ill—a patient is considered to be "dangerously ill" when, based on assessment by a physician or nurse, a patient's illness or condition may be imminently life threatening.

V. PROCEDURES:

A. Department Organization and Staff Responsibilities

1. Personnel

   a. The department is organized with a director, staff clergy, and students in order to meet patient needs for pastoral care.

   b. Chaplains are available to patients and staff according to designated staffing patterns. In addition, *a hospital chaplain is available for emergencies on a twenty-four-hour basis.* The chaplain may be contacted through the hospital switchboard.

   c. The Director of Pastoral Services shall work directly with accredited clinical pastoral training programs to obtain chaplain-interns who provide supervised pastoral care and counseling to the patients.

   d. When appropriate, referrals shall be made to community clergy at the patient's request. All leaders and groups providing religious care or interventions within the hospital shall do so in conjunction with departmental guidelines.

2. Qualifications and Responsibilities of Staff Chaplains

   a. The Director of Pastoral Services and staff chaplains shall be qualified for their positions by education, training, and experience. Chaplain's qualifications are on file in the New Hampshire Hospital Human Resources Department.

   b. The Director of Pastoral Services shall supervise all staff, trainees, and volunteers in accordance with the departmental organization chart.

   c. The Director of Pastoral Services shall ensure pastoral services provided by the hospital are delivered in accordance with written policies and procedures of the department and the hospital.

    d. The Director of Pastoral Services shall chair regularly scheduled departmental meetings and additional meetings as needed.

B. The Scope and Conduct of Pastoral Services

  1. Pastoral Services Provided to Individual Patients

    a. General Visitation
Staff chaplains shall regularly visit patients based on the patient's request, per chaplain visitation schedules, or upon staff or community referrals.

    b. Counseling
(1) Staff chaplains shall be available for counseling on issues pertaining to spiritual needs and as part of the total patient treatment plan.
(2) Regular reviews of this counseling shall take place during departmental meetings and may be noted in the patient's medical record.

    c. Education
(1) The Pastoral Services Department shall provide educational opportunities as appropriate to the spiritual needs of individual patients.

    d. Worship and Devotion
(1) Worship services shall be regularly scheduled.
(2) Individuals who are not able to attend worship services may request sacraments, devotional literature, or may choose to view religious programming on the unit.
(3) Every effort shall be made to provide spiritual direction for one's faith tradition within the resources and limitations of the department and the hospital.

    e. Consultation and Participation in Patient Treatment Plans
(1) As part of a multidisciplinary treatment team, chaplains may participate in patient treatment planning, exceptional occurrence reviews, discussions requiring ethical decision making, and in other related ways.
(2) Consultation with other hospital staff shall be subject to concerns for patient confidentiality, the self-disclosure inherent to pastoral care, and the imminent potential danger of a patient to self or others.

  2. Critical Care Situations of Primary Pastoral Care Concern

    a. Admissions
(1) Newly admitted patients shall be regularly visited based on the patient's request, staff request, or other related referrals.
(2) Daily census movement records shall be obtained by the Pastoral Services Department. This shall include informa-

tion regarding any religious affiliation or preference a patient may have.

(3) All patient requests for a chaplain's visit shall be communicated to the department within one working day.

b. Spiritual Needs Crises

(1) A patient shall be the primary authority when seeking the intervention of a chaplain. All such requests for a chaplain shall be honored.

(2) When it is determined that a patient is experiencing a spiritual needs crisis, a referral shall be made to the Pastoral Services Department.

(3) When the patient is experiencing a spiritual needs crisis and is unable or unwilling to work with a chaplain or a designated consultant, indirect pastoral care may be provided through the treatment team.

c. Dangerously Ill Persons

(1) In order that spiritual needs may be addressed as quickly as possible, Pastoral Services shall be notified when a patient is first determined to be dangerously ill.

(2) The chaplain shall be contacted through the hospital switchboard.

(3) Upon receiving notification that a patient is dangerously ill, a chaplain shall visit the patient as quickly as possible.

(4) When a chaplain responds to an emergency call, a progress note shall be entered in the patient's medical record.

d. Death of a Patient

(1) The Pastoral Services Department shall be notified as soon as possible upon the death of a patient.

(2) The chaplain shall be contacted through the hospital switchboard.

(3) Upon receiving notification that a patient has died, a chaplain shall visit with involved persons as appropriate.

(4) A memorial service shall be held upon the death of a patient. If such a service shall be deemed inappropriate, the chaplain shall consult with the Unit staff to determine other options.

(5) Memorial services shall be held in the chapel, or in any other suitable area for the deceased patient.

(6) Chaplains may participate in services for a deceased patient in places other than at the hospital.

(7) A funeral service shall be conducted by a staff chaplain for all state funerals.

(8) A graveside service shall be conducted by a state chaplain when state facilities are used for burial.

3. Pastoral Services Provided to Patients in Group Settings

When the Department sponsors or cosponsors patient group work, it shall do so with specific goals and objectives which are reviewed and evaluated during regular departmental meetings and are acceptable to the patient and his or her treatment team.

4. Pastoral Services Provided to Patients' Families and Other Visitors

   a. Chaplains shall provide pastoral services to families and visitors based on the patient's request, the chaplain's, or family's initiative or other referrals.
   b. Referrals to outside resources shall be made as appropriate.

5. Pastoral Services Provided to Outside Religious Leaders and Clergy

   a. Religious leaders and clergy shall be invited to educational programs sponsored by the Pastoral Services Department.
   b. The Pastoral Services Department shall provide support and clinical input to religious leaders/clergy at their request.

6. Pastoral Services Provided to Hospital Staff and Trainees

   a. Supportive pastoral care and counseling shall be provided for staff and trainees based on the individual's request, chaplain's initiative, or other referrals.
   b. Referrals to outside resources shall be made as appropriate.
   c. The Pastoral Services Department shall participate in regular training programs for new employees.
   d. The Pastoral Services Department may sponsor educational programs for hospital staff.
   e. The Pastoral Services Department shall participate in joint educational programs and serve on hospital committees as requested or assigned.

7. Pastoral Services Provided to the Community at Large

The Pastoral Services Department shall serve as one of the liaisons between the hospital and the community through programs which foster improved communication concerning mental health issues.

8. Pastoral Services are provided to affiliated on-campus clinical programs in emergency situations.

Revised Date:
This policy applies to: All Services

Appendix E

Sample Pastoral Services Scope of Practice Statement

SERVICE PLAN: Pastoral Services

MISSION: To serve the spiritual needs of patients/residents through quality pastoral care.

CUSTOMERS SERVED: Patients of all ages, family members, interns, wider community, staff based on spiritual need.

MAJOR FUNCTIONS: Provision of worship services, consultation, counseling, pastoral care, education, emergency availability.

ACCESSING SERVICES: Spiritual need assessments, referrals, patient, family, staff request, orientation, chaplain request forms, brochure, team assessments.

ASSESSMENT/SERVICE PLANNING: Some services are provided to all (worship, pastoral care/visitation, memorial services), some are requested (pastoral care, counseling, emergency), and some are referred (therapeutic groups, counseling). Prioritization is based on assessment of need, scheduling, and availability of services and staff. Services reviewed weekly, quarterly, and yearly.

SERVICE MODALITIES/DELIVERY METHODS: One-on-one visitation with patients, families, staff in need; leading of fellowship, conversational, life skill, spiritual care, and recovery groups; participating in orientation-to-unit, morning meeting, and patient and family wellness groups; provision of weekly worship service and memorial services; provision of staff educational programs regarding spiritual needs and grief and loss. Specific response to requests and referrals.

STAFFING: The Pastoral Service Department currently consists of two chaplains who are ordained clergy with specialized training in pastoral care and counseling. Continuing education is provided at a minimum of twenty hours per year and includes departmental, hospital, and other educational opportunities appropriate to our work at the hospital. Work assignments are made by the director of the department and/or collaboratively discussed. Consults from faith traditions in the wider community are referred as needed.

ACCOUNTABILITY STRUCTURES: The director supervises the department personnel including hiring (working with personnel department and the Council of Churches), budget approval (working with business office), and performance evaluation.

COMMUNICATION/ORGANIZATIONAL RELATIONSHIPS: Through staff meetings, supervision, departmental head meetings, team meetings, general consultations, task groups, committees, pastoral care and counseling training of interns and residents, consultation with area clergy and denominations and Council of Churches.

PERFORMANCE EVALUATION: We receive feedback through participant response, patient/family surveys, course evaluations, consultation and team participation, formal suggestions, internal department communication, and evaluation.

ACCOMPLISHMENTS: FY 2000:

Top Three:

1. Availability of Eucharistic Minister for Holy Communion for Catholics
2. Loss and Recovery Group for eldercare patients
3. Developed and distributed winter and summer spiritual care prayer booklets

Other:

4. Revised brochure and chaplain's request form incorporating changes based on patient preferences

GOALS FY 2001:

1. Partners in Wellness Program
2. Children's Family Focus Program
3. Spiritual Care and Recovery Group, Unit D

Chaplain I: Job Description

Classification: _Chaplain I_ **Labor Grade.** **Class Title Code:**

Position Title: _Chaplain I_ **Date Established:**

Position Number: **Date of Last Amendment:**

This position is assigned to work in the support services area.

SCOPE OF WORK:

Provides for the spiritual welfare of the patients/residents of this hospital as a member of the Pastoral Services Department extending to family members, visitors, hospital staff, affiliated clinical program, and to the community at large.

ACCOUNTABILITIES:

- Provides for a variety of religious services for patients/residents and staff to enrich their spiritual heritage and traditions.

- Visits, counsels, and refers patients/residents to nurture and support their spiritual growth and development.

- Develops educational programs and resources to inform, support, and train patients/residents and staff.

- Coordinates volunteer religious activities and supervises the assisting volunteers to make available a larger number of outside resources.

- Gathers and presents information from pastoral care and counseling sessions to coordinate therapy and religious counseling goals in a multidisciplinary team treatment process.

- Serves on committees and develops educational, recreational, or clinical programs for patient/residents as a member of the hospital staff.

MINIMUM QUALIFICATIONS:

- See Class Specification for Chaplain I.

SPECIAL QUALIFICATIONS:

- Ordination as a minister, priest, or rabbi in a recognized faith tradition (denomination) and ecclesiastically endorsed by that denomination (in good standing).

DISCLAIMER STATEMENT: The supplemental job description lists typical examples of work and is not intended to include every job duty and responsibility specific to a position. An employee may be required to perform other related duties not listed on the supplemental job description provided that such duties are characteristic of that classification.

SIGNATURES:

Appendix G

Chaplain II: Clinical Education Coordinator/Director Job Description

Classification: __Chaplain II__   Labor Grade. Class Title Code:

Position Title: __Chaplain II__   Date Established:

Position Number: Date of Last Amendment:

This position is assigned to work with the adult, child/adolescent, geriatric psychiatric client population.

SCOPE OF WORK:

Responds to the spiritual needs of the patients/residents of this hospital through quality pastoral care as a chaplain in the Department of Pastoral Services and directs the clinical pastoral education training program and/or the counseling intern training program. Services are provided, in addition and as appropriate, to family members, visitors, hospital staff, affiliated clinical programs, and to the community at large.

ACCOUNTABILITIES:

- Coordinates the clinical pastoral education program at this hospital to meet the accreditation standards of the Theological School Cluster and the Association of Clinical Pastoral Educators. AND/OR Coordinates the counseling training program to meet the standards of the American Association of Pastoral Counselors.

- Directs the clinical pastoral training program(s) and plans cooperatively with the Director of Pastoral Services, the Department of Pastoral Services, hospital department heads, unit directors, and others as appropriate to ensure that programs and services benefit the patients/residents.

279

- Supervises all trainees in the clinical pastoral program(s) to maintain quality pastoral care, counseling, and worship services to the patients/residents.

- Visits, counsels, and consults as a member of the multidisciplinary treatment team to nurture and support the spiritual growth and development of patients/residents.

- Plans, leads, and provides worship services, rites, and rituals for patients/residents and staff to respond to people's spiritual needs and rights to religious expression.

- Develops educational programs and resources to inform, support, and train patients/residents, staff, clergy, seminarians, and laypersons.

- Presents solutions and goals to community religious and related groups to offer guidance in establishing a favorable environment for those returning to the community.

MINIMUM QUALIFICATIONS:

- See Class Specification for Chaplain II

LICENSE/CERTIFICATION:

- Certified Educator/Supervisor in American Association of Clinical Pastoral Education or in American Association of Pastoral Counselors or equivalents.

DISCLAIMER STATEMENT: The supplemental job description lists typical examples of work and is not intended to include every job duty and responsibility specific to a position. An employee may be required to perform other related duties not listed on the supplemental job description provided that such duties are characteristic of that classification.

SIGNATURES:

Appendix H

Chaplain IV: Administrator/Director Job Description

Classification: _Chaplain IV_   **Labor Grade:**   **Class Title Code:**

Position Title: _ADMINISTRATOR/DIRECTOR_   **Date Established:**

Position Number: **Date of Last Amendment:**

This position is assigned to work with the adult, child/adolescent, and geriatric psychiatric client population.

SCOPE OF WORK:

Directs and administers the Pastoral Services Department of this hospital so as to serve the spiritual needs of the patients/residents of the hospital through quality pastoral care. This service extends to family members, visitors, hospital staff, affiliated on campus clinical programs, and to the community at large.

ACCOUNTABILITIES:

- Provides for, supervises, and evaluates the clinical services and religious programs within the Department of Pastoral Services to meet the policies and procedures of the department and the hospital, and to provide quality pastoral care.

- Supervises and evaluates the functioning of chaplains and other personnel within the department to ensure quality pastoral care/services and to meet review standards of the hospital.

- Provides for the clinical pastoral training center, and the training program for pastoral counseling interns and residents, to ensure that the center/program meets the national accreditation standards and functions within the department and as part of the hospital.

- Advises and counsels patients/residents and staff on spiritual needs or closely related issues to provide support and therapeutic counseling services.

- Participates in diagnostic and staff conferences to provide therapeutic services as part of a multidisciplinary team.

- Conducts a variety of religious services and programs for patients/residents and employees to provide for the spiritual needs and traditions of persons at the hospital.

- Plans and directs religious volunteer activities to provide a wider range of resources for patients/residents.

- Presents solutions and goals to community religious and related groups to offer guidance in establishing a favorable environment for those returning to the community.

MINIMUM QUALIFICATIONS:

- See Class Specification for CHAPLAIN IV

DISCLAIMER STATEMENT: The supplemental job description lists typical examples of work and is not intended to include every job duty and responsibility specific to a position. An employee may be required to perform other related duties not listed on the supplemental job description provided that such duties are characteristic of that classification.

SIGNATURES:

Appendix I
Sample Brochure

CLINICAL PASTORAL EDUCATION

"CPE" Chaplains and students:

are ordained clergy or studying for the ministry.

come from many faith traditions.

seek to spend time in supervised ministry at Beverly Hospital and Addison Gilbert Hospital

are assigned to the buildings and associated facilities of Northeast Health Systems.

are involved in worship services, relationship, fellowship, friendship and Bible Studies.

are always under the supervision of the Chaplaincy Director.

End of Life and Ethical issues

Often the suddenness of illness and the complexity of medical technology confronts patients and their loved ones with difficult decisions. The hospital chaplain has a long tradition of moral guidance to help with the issues that arise in "end of life" situations.

The Health Care Proxy is one important preparation. Patients are encouraged to speak with family members, their primary care physician, pastoral ministers, and others to discuss their values, convictions, and possible decisions. The proxy is an individual who is appointed in writing to act in case of emergency, when the patient is unable to do so.

Faith tradition values life from the moment of conception through the moment of natural death. It encourages appropriate measures for the relief of pain and does not feel it is necessary to prolong the dying process with the unlimited use of medical interventions. Pastoral services are available to support and assist the terminally ill person and his/her family, in finding comfort, meaning and strength.

Chaplaincy Services
at

Addison Gilbert Hospital & Beverly Hospital

Affiliates of Northeast Health Systems Inc.

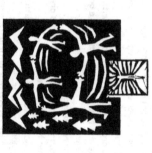

The Northeast Health Systems Chaplaincy Department is directed by Rev. John C. Pearson, D.Min., who is a Diplomate with the American Association of Pastoral Counselors and a Supervisor of Clinical Pastoral Education
(978) 922, ext. 2791
or page through the operator

283

A HEALTH CARE CHAPLAIN IS

an ordained priest, minister, rabbi or trained lay person, who chooses to minister to people in places like: Beverly Hospital, Addison Gilbert Hospital, BayRidge Hospital, Cable Emergency Center, The Hunt Center, CAB Health & Recovery Services, Inc., Family Practice Center, Heritage at Danvers, The Herrick House, Ledgewood Rehabilitation and Skilled Nursing Center, North Shore Birth Center, North Shore Rehabilitation and Skilled Nursing Center, and Seacoast Nursing and Retirement Center.

The Addison Gilbert and Beverly Hospital Clinical Pastoral Education Program is accredited by:

The Association for Clinical Pastoral Education, Inc.
549 Clairmont Road, Suite 103
Decatur, Georgia 30033
(404) 320-1472
and the U.S. Department of Education

PASTORAL SERVICES OFFER

- PASTORAL CARE AND COUNSELING to clients, residents and staff WORSHIP, prayer, meditation, Communion and confession.

- PASTORAL CARE through conversation, relationship, fellowship and friendship. COUNSELING to help people find integration, wholeness and health by focusing on specific life issues.

- SPIRITUAL DIRECTION by being open to beliefs and actions of the heart and of the world.

- EDUCATION through individual and small group programs offered during the course of the year.

EXAMPLES OF WHEN YOU MIGHT WANT TO SEE A CHAPLAIN:

You are feeling anxious, lonely or isolated.
You are concerned about family, loved ones or yourself.
You desire prayer or confession.
You are experiencing an emotional and/or spiritual crisis.
You are having difficulty coping with your stay and feel a chaplain could be a good listener.
You are feeling guilty.
When you are feeling that things aren't going the way you wish.
You have questions about your faith or religion.
You have received or anticipate some bad news.
You have questions about Pastoral Services and how ministry affects you during your stay.
You desire to receive sacraments and are unable to attend worship.
You feel like celebrating: you're going home, you're feeling better, and you've had a good week!

Appendix J

Identifying Professional Needs

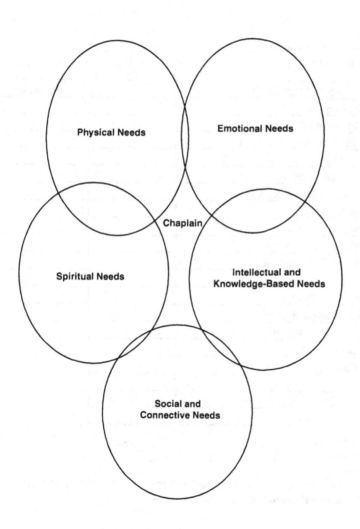

Physical Needs

Emotional Needs

Chaplain

Spiritual Needs

Intellectual and
Knowledge-Based Needs

Social and
Connective Needs

Appendix K

Department of Pastoral Services Sample Orientation Checklist

Orientation for: _____

Date of Hire: _____ Assignment: _____

KNOWLEDGE OF:		INITIALS
Work Assignment		
Departmental Activities		
Intro Spiritual Needs/Resources		
Intro Loss and Recovery		
Departmental Compentencies		
Pastoral Services Policy & Manual		
Professional Ethics		
Continuing Education		
Quality Assurance Activities		
Treatment Plans and Teams		
Documentation Requirements		
Clinical Case Review		
Confidentiality and Chaplains		
Hospital Policy Manual Location		
Mental Health System		
Age-Specific Orientation:		
Adults		
Children and Youth		
Geropsych		

Employee _____

Director _____

Date: _____

Applies to student/interns unless otherwise indicated by Director

Return to Director of Pastoral Services

PART 2: PASTORAL SERVICES

NAME:

ORIENTATION DATE:_____DATE OF COMPLETION:_____

1. All components of this checklist shall be attended. Once a section is completed, it shall be signed with your full name and title of presenter.
2. This orientation is to be completed during the first two weeks of your rotation.
3. Once completed, the original form shall be returned to the Director of Pastoral Services.
4. This orientation is a requirement by hospital policy.

PROCEDURE	DATE	PRESENTER	SIGNATURE/PRESENTER
REHABILITATION SERVICES			
COMMUNITY INTEGRATION			
QUALITY ASSURANCE			
STAFF DEVELOPMENT			
DIR OF NURSING			
MEDICAL INFORMATION			
TRANSITIONAL HOUSING SERVICES			
PSYCHOLOGY			
ASSISSTANT SUPERINTENDENT			
SUPERINTENDENT			

I have met with staff presenters on this checklist and understand the policies, procedures, and information discussed with them.

Signature: _____   Date: _____

Appendix L
Spiritual Needs Assessment

Rate each item from 1-5 with 1 being at the low end of the continuum and 5 at the high end. Rate each item to the best of your ability. When you have finished, add up the numbers in each area and place in the subtotal below that section. For those who are using this form as a way to assess the spiritual needs of others, you would ask the person about each area and fill in your assessment on the form.

PHILOSOPHY OF LIFE	no	undecided		think so	yes
I know my likes and dislikes	1	2	3	4	5
I have some control over my life and behavior	1	2	3	4	5
I am aware of my beliefs and values	1	2	3	4	5
I see meaning in life and my illness does make sense to me	1	2	3	4	5

subtotal_____

SENSE OF HOPE	no	undecided		think so	yes
I often feel hopeful	1	2	3	4	5
I can say "yes" to life	1	2	3	4	5
I see the world as a friendly place	1	2	3	4	5
My life can get better	1	2	3	4	5

subtotal_____

CONCEPT OF GOD OR HIGHER POWER	no	undecided		think so	yes
I know that God cares about me	1	2	3	4	5
I have religious/spiritual practices that are important to me	1	2	3	4	5
I am aware of spiritual doubts and conflicts	1	2	3	4	5
I know kindness/grace in my own life	1	2	3	4	5

subtotal_____

CONNECTIONS TO THE WORLD

CONNECTIONS TO THE WORLD	no	undecided		think so	yes
I have friends	1	2	3	4	5
I feel a part of a group (family, town, set of people)	1	2	3	4	5
I am connected to a tradition (Polish, Lutheran, Catholic, Democrat or Republican)	1	2	3	4	5
I feel close to nature	1	2	3	4	5

subtotal_____

SELF-FULFILLMENT	no	undecided		think so	yes
I have gifts and talents	1	2	3	4	5
I have creative moments	1	2	3	4	5
I know what seems beautiful to me	1	2	3	4	5
I have positive ways of meeting my own spiritual needs	1	2	3	4	5

subtotal_____

Key to Spiritual Needs Assessment:
A low score (4-6) in any one of the five areas may indicate spiritual distress and a need for help in that area.

A high score (16-20) in any one of the five areas may indicate that that area is a spiritual care resource and can be drawn on when other areas are currently in distress.

Note: A person may believe in God or a Higer Power, in which case substitute the belief focus (humanity, family, the goddess).

Appendix M

Care Readiness Questionnaire

DIRECTIONS: The questions below represent the phases and key processes that are a part of readiness to engage in hospital ministry. Go through each area and ask yourself: Is this true of me? Pencil in a YES, NO, or MAYBE. Remember that those engaged in hospital ministry cycle through these phases and processes, to some degree, throughout their ministry.

Contemplation

I am aware that there is a need for persons to minister to those who are ill and hospitalized.
I have had experiences visiting those who are ill and hospitalized.
I think that I am the type of person who could minister to those who are ill and hospitalized.
I believe that I am called to hospital ministry.

Preparation

I am willing to go to school to learn how to minister to those who are ill and hospitalized.
I am willing to practice ministering to those who are ill and hospitalized and to receive clinical training in this ministry.
I find that I really want to do this kind of ministry.
I have made some contacts with schools and hospitals that provide clinical pastoral training. I have spoken with persons already engaged in hospital ministry, so I have a sense of what I have to do.

Action

As I engage in hospital ministry I find that I am usually aware of the needs of others.
I can identify the pastoral care and counseling services that I am skilled at providing.

I find that I am able to think, plan, and act with a sense of knowing what I am doing.

I accept that God is connected with my ministry. At times, I can understand some of these connections.

Reflection

I believe that I know what I am doing and can reflect on my ministry in ways that help me to do better.

I find that I am learning all the time. I am therefore able to identify skills that I want to develop further.

I feel good about what I do and am motivated to continue this work.

I can see how hospital ministry is what I am called to do. Therefore, I feel connected with others in the field, with God, and am at peace within myself.

Appendix N

Religious Preference Codes

SAMPLE 1: NEW HAMPSHIRE HOSPITAL

**FIELD #9—Religion

10 = JEWISH
11 = ROMAN CATHOLIC
12 = GREEK ORTHODOX
13 = EPISCOPAL
14 = LUTHERAN
15 = CONGREGATIONAL
16 = BAPTIST
17 = METHODIST
18 = CHRISTIAN SCIENCE
19 = PROTESTANT
20 = CHRISTIAN
21 = JEHOVAH'S WITNESS
22 = MORMON
23 = NONE
98 = OTHER
99 = UNKNOWN

SAMPLE 2: MASSACHUSETTS GENERAL HOSPITAL

AC   ADVENT CHRISTIAN
AG   AGNOSTIC
AN   ANGLICAN
AT   ATHEIST
BA   BAHAI

BP BAPTIST
BU BUDDHIST
CH CHRISTIAN
CN DISCIPLES OF CHRIST
CO CONGREGATIONAL
DE DEFERRED
EC EVANGELICAL CONGREGATIONAL
EP EPISCOPAL
HE JEWISH
LU LUTHERAN
MO MORMON
MS MUSLIM
MT METHODIST
NA NOT AFFILIATED
NP NO PREFERENCE
OR ORTHODOX
OT OTHER
PN PENTECOSTAL
PR PROTESTANT
PT PRESBYTERIAN
RC ROMAN CATHOLIC
SB SOUTHERN BAPTIST
SD SEVENTH-DAY ADVENTIST
SP SPIRITUALIST
UN UNKNOWN
UU UNITARIAN-UNIVERSALIST
WI WICCAN

Appendix O

Typical Presenting Problems: Brief Counseling

Emergency and Cardiac Care

Shock and trauma
Anger
Punishment from God
Grief and loss

Kidney Dialysis

Grief and loss
Living with a chronic illness
End of life issues

Maternity

Family education
Adjustment to changes a child brings
Couple treatment

Medical Surgical

Pain management
Lifestyle changes
Stress reduction

Pediatrics

Family dynamics
Management of fear and helplessness
Education of treatment choices

Psychiatric

    Grief, loss, and recovery
    Managing mental illness
    Spiritual resources and practices
    Anger with God
    Family and relationships
    Trauma and recovery

Staff Support

    Issues for the "working poor"
    Burnout and stress on the job
    Theological issues about workplace values
    Personal and family issues
    Anxiety, depression, personality conflicts with co-worker or boss

Substance abuse

    Lifestyle choices
    Faith in God/higher power
    Loss and recovery

Appendix P

Introduction to Supervision: Pre–Self-Assessment

Name:
Date:

Please rate the following:	Agree	Somewhat Agree	Somewhat Disagree	Disagree
I have a clear understanding of what it means to be a supervisor.	4	3	2	1
I frequently give sincere and specific feedback to my supervisees.	4	3	2	1
I frequently listen to my supervisees.	4	3	2	1
I frequently share my thoughts, feelings, and rationale with my supervisees.	4	3	2	1
I encourage involvement in projects and decision making with my supervisees.	4	3	2	1
I give support to my supervisees without taking on their assignments.	4	3	2	1
I have an awareness of some ethical dilemmas that occur in my work area. (see below)	4	3	2	1
I feel comfortable in working to resolve an ethical dilemma in my work area.	4	3	2	1

Note: An ethical dilemma can be defined as a situation that involves a choice between two or more courses of action. The situation usually involves conflicting values.

Appendix Q

Introduction to Supervision: Post–Self-Assessment

This assessment will not impact your participation in the program in any way, nor will it be shared with your supervisor. It is soley for the purpose of helping us determine whether this program was effective. Please be as honest as possible.

Name: Date:

Please rate the following:	Agree	Somewhat Agree	Somewat Disagree	Disagree
I have a clear understanding of what it means to be a supervisor.	4	3	2	1
I frequently give sincere and specific feedback to my supervisees.	4	3	2	1
I frequently listen to my supervisees.	4	3	2	1
I frequently share my thoughts, feelings, and rationale with my supervisees.	4	3	2	1
I encourage involvement in projects and decision making with my supervisees.	4	3	2	1
I give support to my supervisees without taking on their assignments.	4	3	2	1
I have an awareness of some ethical dilemmas that occur in my work area. (see below)	4	3	2	1
I feel comfortable in working to resolve an ethical dilemma in my work area.	4	3	2	1

In the past week, I have used the knowledge and skills from this program in the following way(s):

Appendix R

Sample of Group Referral Form

PATIENT REFERRAL FOR PASTORAL SERVICES GROUPS

Patient Name: Date:

Referring Team: Patient #:

                                                 Treatment Code#:

                                                 Diagnosis:

Referred To (add or subtract from list to fit needs)
  —Conversations with the Chaplains
  —Spirituality and Recovery
  —Grief, Loss, and Recovery
  —Lifestyle Choices
  —Trauma Recovery

Reason for Referral: (brief background and goals)

Known Risk Factors: (add or substract from basic list to fit needs)
  —Substance abuse/dependence
  —Medication noncompliance
  —Question of physical or sexual abuse
  —Symptoms related to diagnosis are stabilizing
  —Relationship difficulties
  —Suicidal ideation
  —Homicidal ideation
  —Potential for self-abuse
  —Assuasive behavior
  —Awol risk

Appendix S

Sample Group Documentation Log

Leland Unit/PHP
Group Documentation Log

	Attendance	Self-Assessment
Date Time Group Name: Material Covered:	[ ] Yes [ ] No [ ] Excused [ ] Left early [ ] Came late [ ] Not group app. [ ] Too late for group Comments:	[ ] Spontaneous conversation [ ] Needed prompting [ ] No participation [ ] Good focus [ ] Poor focus [ ] Intermittent focus [ ] Disorganized thoughts [ ] Disorganized task skills [ ] Organized [ ] Appropriate interactions [ ] Intrusive behavior [ ] Impulsive behavior [ ] Responsive to limit setting Y N [ ] Reports suicidal ideation Y N [ ] Reports homicidal ideation Y N Insight into illness Good Fair Poor Group Leader:

Bibliography

American Heritage Dictionary of the English Language, The (1973). Boston: Houghton Mifflin.

Beck, Cornelia, Ruth Rawlins, and Sophronia Williams (1988). *Mental Health-Psychiatric Nursing: A Holistic Life-Cycle Approach*, Second Edition. St. Louis: C.V. Mosby.

Beckhard, Richard and Wendy Pritchard (1992). *Changing the Essence: The Art of Creating and Leading Fundamental Change in Organizations*. San Francisco: Jossey-Bass.

Belgum, David (1999). "Dealing with Cultural Diversity: A Hospital Chaplain Reflects on Gypsies and Other Such Diversity." *The Journal of Pastoral Care, 53*(2): 175-181.

Bellandi, Deanna (2000). "A Prayerful Experience, Hospital Chaplains Are There to Help Patients at Most-Vulnerable Moments." *Modern Healthcare*, July 24: 14-16.

Bennis, Warren and Joan Goldsmith (1994). *Learning to Lead: A Workbook on Becoming a Leader*. Reading, MA: Addison-Wesley.

Benson, Herbert (1996). *Timeless Healing: The Power and Biology of Belief*. New York: Scribner.

Billman, Kathleen D. (1996)."Pastoral Care As an Art of Community," Christie Cozad Neuger (Ed.), *The Arts of Ministry: Feminist-Womanist Approaches* (pp. 10-38). Louisville, KY: Westminster John Knox Press.

Block, Peter (1993). *Stewardship: Choosing Service Over Self-Interest*. San Francisco: Berrett-Koehler.

Boie, Eric, Gregory P. Moore, Chad Brummett, and David R. Nelson (1999). "Do Parents Want to Be Present During Invasive Procedures Performed on Their Children in the Emergency Department? A Survey of 400 Parents." *Annals of Emergency Medicine, 34*(1): 70-74.

Borg, Marcus (1998). *The God We Never Knew*. San Francisco: HarperSanFrancisco.

Bussema, Kenneth and Evelyn Bussema (2000). "Is There a Balm in Gilead? The Implications of Faith in Coping with a Psychiatric Disability." *Psychiatric Rehabilitation Journal, 24*(2): 117-124.

Capps, Donald (1997). "The Letting Loose of Hope: Where Psychology of Religion and Pastoral Care Converge." *The Journal of Pastoral Care, 51*(2): 139-149.

Carmel, Sara (1999). "Life-Sustaining Treatments: What Doctors Do, What They Want for Themselves and What Elderly Persons Want." *Social Science and Medicine, 49:* 1401-1408.

Cheston, Sharon E. and Robert J. Wicks (1993). *Essentials for Chaplains.* New York: Paulist Press.

Covey, Stephen (1990). *The 7 Habits of Highly Effective People.* New York: Simon and Schuster.

Dossey, Larry (1993). *Healing Words: The Power of Prayer and the Practice of Medicine.* New York: HarperCollins.

Ehman, John W, Barbara B. Ott, Thomas H. Short, Ralph C. Ciampa, and John Hansen-Flaschen (1999). "Do Patients Want Physicians to Inquire About Their Spiritual or Religious Beliefs if They Become Gravely Ill?" *Archives of Internal Medicine, 159*(15): 1803-1806.

Engstrom, Susan and Diane Madlon-Kay (1998). "Choosing a Family Physician: What Do Patients Want to Know?" *Minnesota Medicine, 81:* 22-26.

Evans, Abigail Rian (1999). *Redeeming Marketplace Medicine: A Theology of Health Care.* Cleveland: The Pilgrim Press.

Feldman-Stewart, Deb, Michael D. Brundage, Charles Hayter, Patti Groome, J. Curtis Nickel, Heather Downes, and William J. Mackillop (2000). "What Questions Do Patients with Curable Prostate Cancer Want Answered?" *Medical Decision Making, 29*(1): 7-19.

Gerkin, Charles (1984). *The Living Human Document: Re-Visioning Pastoral Counseling in a Hermeneutical Mode.* Nashville: Abingdon Press.

Gibbons, Graeme, Andrew Retsas, and Jaya Pinkahana (1999). "Describing What Chaplains Do in Hospitals," *The Journal of Pastoral Care, 53*(2): 201-207.

Groll, Richard, Michael Wensing, Jan Mainz, Pedro Ferreira, Hilary Hearnshaw, Per Hjortdahl, Frede Olesen, Mats Ribacke, Tomi Spenser, and Joachim Szecseny (1999). "Patients' Priorities with Respect to General Practice Care: An International Comparison," *Family Practice, 16*(1): 4-11.

Halverson, Delia (1999). *The Gift of Hospitality.* St. Louis: Chalice Press.

Hoencamp, Erik (1999)."Yes, Doctor, No, Doctor: What Do Patients Want From You?," Editorial, *Acta Psychiactric Scandinavia, 100:* 319-320.

Holy Bible, The (1971). Revised Standard Version (RSV), Second Edition. Nashville: Thomas Nelson, Inc.

Jones, Laurie Beth (1995). *Jesus CEO: Using Ancient Wisdom for Visionary Leadership.* New York: Hyperion.

Kari, Jameela A, Chris Donnovan, Jun Li, and Brent Taylor (1999). "Teenagers in Hospital: What Do They Want?" *Nursing Standard, 13*(23): 49-51.

Kestenbaum, Rabbi Israel (1997). "A Jewish Approach to Healing." *The Journal of Pastoral Care, 51*(2): 207-211.

Kim, Michael K, and Aijaz Alvi (1999). "Breaking the Bad News of Cancer: The Patient's Perspective." *Laryngoscope, 109:* 1064-1067.

Kirkwood, Nevelle A. (1998). *Pastoral Care in Hospitals.* Harrisburg, PA: More-house Publishing.

Koenig, Harold (1997). *Is Religion Good for Your Health?* Binghamton, NY: The Haworth Pastoral Press.

Kornfeld, Margaret (1998). *Cultivating Wholeness: A Guide to Care and Counseling in Faith Communities.* New York: Continuum.

Lester, Andrew D. (1995). *Hope in Pastoral Care and Counseling.* Louisville, KY: Westminster John Knox Press.

MacPherson, Cluny (1985). "Samoan Medicine." In Clair D. F. Parsons (Ed.), *Healing Practices in the South Pacific* (pp. 1-15). Honolulu: The Institute for Polynesian Studies.

McCall, Junietta Baker (1999). *Grief Education for Caregivers of the Elderly.* Binghamton, NY: The Haworth Pastoral Press.

Moessner, Jeanne Stevenson (Ed.) (1996). *Through the Eyes of Women: Insights for Pastoral Care.* Minneapolis: Fortress Press.

Moller, Mary D. (1999). "Meeting Spiritual Needs on an Inpatient Unit." *Journal of Psychosocial Nursing, 37*(11): 5-10.

Muller, Wayne (1996) *How, Then, Shall We Live?* New York: Bantam.

Noble, L.M, B.C. Douglas, and S.P. Newman (1999). "What Do Patients Want and Do We Want to Know? A Review of Patients' Requests of Psychiatric Services." *Acta Psychiatric Scandinavia, 100:* 321-327.

Nolan, Timothy, Leonard Goodstein, and J. William Pfeiffer (1993). *Plan or Die! 10 Keys to Organizational Success.* San Diego: Pfeiffer and Company.

Oliver, Mary (1994). *A Poetry Handbook.* New York: Harcourt Brace and Company.

Pastoral Care Week Committee FY 2000, P.O. Box 070473, Milwaukee, WI 53207-0473.

Peale, Norman Vincent (1996). *The Power of Positive Thinking.* Reissue. New York: Ballantine.

Poyatos, Fernando (1999). *I Was Sick and You Visited Me: A Spiritual Guide for Catholics in Hospital Ministry.* New York: Paulist Press.

Prochaska, James, John Norcross, and Carlo DiClemente (1994). *Changing for Good,* First Edition. New York: William Morrow and Company, Inc.

Purvis-Smith, Terry A. (1997). "Pastoral Care of the Premature Baby." *The Journal of Pastoral Care, 51*(1): 49-56.

Richardson, Robert L. (2000). "Where There Is Hope, There Is Life: Toward a Biology of Hope." *The Journal of Pastoral Care, 54*(1): 75-83.

Roberts, Jan (2000). Supervisory Development Program, New Hampshire Hospital, Concord, NH.

Rodriguez, Jesus (1999). "Chaplains' Communications with Latino Patients: Case Studies on Nonverbal Communication." *The Journal of Pastoral Care, 53*(3): 309-317.

Ryan, M. J. (1994). *A Grateful Heart: Daily Blessings for the Evening Meal from Buddha to the Beatles.* Berkeley, CA: Conari Press.

Schaper, Donna (1995). *Teaching My Daughter to Mulch: Gardening Meditations.* South Deerfield, MA: Ash Grove Press.

Schlauch, Chris (1995). *Faithful Companioning: How Pastoral Counseling Heals.* Minneapolis: Fortress Press.

Senge, Peter, Art Kleiner, Charlotte Roberts, Richard Ross, and Brian Smith (1994). *The Fifth Discipline Fieldbook: Strategies and Tools for Building a Learning Organization.* New York: Currency, Doubleday.

Simmonds, Anne L. (1997). "Pastoral Perspectives in Intensive Care: Experiences of Doctors and Nurses with Dying Patients." *The Journal of Pastoral Care, 51*(3): 271-281.

Sims, C. Leon (1998). "Toward a Postmodern Chaplaincy." *The Journal of Pastoral Care, 52*(3): 249-259.

Stanley, Andrea (2000). Educational Resources: First-Step Program, Beverly Hospital, Beverly, MA. Results from Picker Survey, March 7.

Stern, Chaim (Ed.) (1982). *Gates of Prayer: The New Union Prayerbook.* New York: Central Conference of American Rabbis.

Stokes, Janet (1999). "Ministry of Presence and Presence of the Spirit in Pastoral Visitation." *The Journal of Pastoral Care, 53*(2): 191-199.

TenBrook, Gretchen (2000). *Broken Bodies, Healing Hearts: Reflections of a Hospital Chaplain.* Binghamton, NY: The Haworth Pastoral Press.

Thurman, Howard (Reprint, 1953). *Meditations of the Heart.* Richmond, IN: Harper and Row.

VandeCreek, Larry (1999a). "Professional Chaplaincy: An Absent Profession?" *The Journal of Pastoral Care, 53*(4): 417-432.

VandeCreek, Larry (1999b). "The Unique Benefits of Religious Support During Cardiac Bypass Surgery." *The Journal of Pastoral Care, 53*(1): 19-29.

VandeCreek, Larry and Stephanie Gibson (1997). "Religious Support from Parish Clergy for Hospitalized Parishioners: Availability, Evaluation, Implications." *The Journal of Pastoral Care, 51*(4): 403-414.

Webster's New Ideal Dictionary (1978). USA: G. and C. Merriam.

Wheatley, Margaret J. (1999). *Leadership and the New Science: Discovering Order in a Chaotic World.* San Francisco: Berrett-Koehler Publishers.

Index

Mercy Hospital customer service
   review, 53-54
Merrimack Association of the United
   Church of Christ, 169
Miller-McLemore, Bonnie, 170
Mind, body, and spirit connection,
   16-17, 80-81, 247-248
Ministry in hospital settings, 20, 23,
   43-44
   field challenges and changes, 36-43
   ministry profile, 115-117
   newer traditions, 23, 25-27, 31-34
   recent directions, 23, 28, 34-35
   traditional ministries, 23, 24, 28-30
   values in ministry, 112-115
Mission for ministry, 21, 105. *See also*
   Values; Vision for ministry
   age-specific considerations, 130
   assumptions, 105-107
   diversity of spirituality, styles,
      and traditions, 129-130
   inclusivity, 130-131
   mission statement
      creation, 127-128
      defined, 124
      examples, 127
   models, 124-127
      holistic healing, 126-127
      salvation and witness, 125-126
      visitation and comfort, 126
   practicing, 131-132
   scope of practice, 131-132
Mission-mandate fulfilled, 15-16
Models
   caring context for health
      and healing, 162
   mechanistic, 76
   mission-based hospital ministry,
      124-127
      holistic healing, 126-127
      salvation and witness, 125-126
      visitation and comfort, 126
   Self-in-Relation, 243
   vision-based hospital ministry,
      119-121
      Babylon captivity vision, 121

Models *(continued)*
   complementary visions, 120-121
   responsible stewardship vision-
      setting, 120
   single shared vision, 120
Moessner, Jeanne Stevenson, 169, 170
Muller, Wayne, 133
Multiple contexts, involvement in,
   17-18
Multiple imagery constellations, 98

National Association of Catholic
   Chaplains, 150
Nearing, Helen, 16
Nebulous imagery and loose
   representations, 97-98
Needs of hospital ministry, 11
   church integration, 13-14, 42-43
   community integration, 14
   link with other spiritual traditions,
      14-15
   paradigm value shift, 11-12
   systems integration and advocacy,
      13
   training and education, 12, 248-249
Networking needs of persons in
   hospital ministry, 135, 137,
   146-150
New Hampshire Hospital
   Catholic chaplain, 38
   diversity of spirituality, styles,
      and traditions, 129-130
   focus groups, 64-67
   history of chaplain services, 29-30,
      38
   history of integration within
      churches, 13-14
   holistic dimensions of personhood,
      135-136, 165
   length of stay on average, 50
   nursing students' psychiatric
      rotation, 261-262
   paradigm value shift, 11-12
   self-improvement, 105
   spiritual care request form, 59-60

Printed in the United States
by Baker & Taylor Publisher Services